Brief Strategic Therapy

Brief Strategic Therapy

Philosophy, Techniques, and Research

GIORGIO NARDONE
AND
PAUL WATZLAWICK

JASON ARONSON

Lanham • Boulder • New York • Toronto • Oxford

Published in the United States of America
by Jason Aronson
An imprint of Rowman & Littlefield Publishers, Inc.

A wholly owned subsidiary of
The Rowman & Littlefield Publishing Group, Inc.
4501 Forbes Boulevard, Suite 200, Lanham, Maryland 20706
www.rowmanlittlefield.com

PO Box 317
Oxford
OX2 9RU, UK

This book was set in 12 pt. Bembo by Alpha Graphics of Pittsfield, NH, and printed and
bound by Book-mart Press, Inc. of North Bergen, NJ.

British Library Cataloguing in Publication Information Available
Library of Congress Cataloging-in-Publication Data

Nardone, Giorgio.
    Brief strategic therapy / Giorgio Nardone, Paul Watzlawick.
        p. cm.
    Includes bibliographical references and index.
    ISBN 0-7657-0280-0
    1. Strategic therapy. 2. Brief psychotherapy. I. Watzlawick, Paul. II. Title.
RC489.S76 N373 2000
616.89'14—dc21   00-056939

Printed in the United States of America

⊖™ The paper used in this publication meets the minimum requirements of American
National Standard for Information Sciences—Permanence of Paper for Printed Library
Materials, ANSI/NISO Z39.48-1992.

Contents

Introduction

I take great pleasure in introducing a book that I consider to be an important contribution to the field of what is now known as brief strategic therapy or, more precisely, the practical application of radical constructivism, systems theory, and the concept of self-organization to human problems.

Giorgio Nardone and I met many years ago when I supervised part of his intensive training at the Brief Therapy Center in the Mental Research Institute of Palo Alto, California, of which I am a member. Since then we have remained in contact, and I have thus been able to observe and participate in the establishment and growth of his Center for Strategic Therapy (Centro di Terapia Strategica in Arezzo, Italy). Together we have held seminars and conferences all around the world in which we have presented the interactional (as opposed to the classical individual, retrospective, and analytical) view of problem formation and problem resolution to clinicians as well as to managers of large organizations.

This book presents a detailed account of Nardone's techniques and of the specific interventions that he has developed, especially in his work with clients suffering from anxiety, phobias, obsessive-compulsive problems, and eating disorders. It ends with a detailed survey and evaluation of the results obtained by these techniques. It is not, therefore, just a "cookbook" giving a superficial description of general guidelines, but rather a detailed account of both the theory and the application of this method of dealing with human problems.

THE BRIEF STRATEGIC
THERAPY APPROACH

The considerable difference between the function of the therapist who employs strategic methods and that of the traditional psychotherapist can be made clearer by comparing the strategic approach to the game of chess. First, just as in a manual of chess, the rules of the game are given, together with the usual procedure from the first move to the checkmate. Subsequently, a series of effective moves and strategies are described. Finally, we are shown a few unusual games that illustrate how, by the interaction of moves and countermoves, the tactics of the game become extremely complex. The limitation of this analogy is that, unlike chess, therapy is not a zero-sum game, that is, a game in which there is usually a winner and a loser. Rather, the game ends with both players (therapist and patient) sharing the win or the loss. By implication, then, any means used by strategic therapists in trying to win their and their patients' games take on a deep ethical value, even when they appear to be deliberately manipulative, because the aim is to find a rapid, effective solution to each patient's problems. When this is borne in mind, the accusation that traditional psychotherapists frequently make, that strategic therapists are treacherous manipulators, becomes devoid of meaning.

OVERVIEW OF THE CONTENTS

Chapter 1 presents the recent developments in the field of psychotherapy and defines the theoretical and practical features that distinguish the strategic method from others.

Chapter 2 explains the type of nonordinary mathematical logic underlying advanced brief strategic therapy techniques, showing that apparently simple techniques are based on a complex and well-constructed logic of intervention.

Chapter 3 explains the basic conceptual characteristics of this method (hereafter referred to as "heresies" because they question the traditional "truths" of psychotherapy). They are the systemic, constructivist basis; a specific theory of persistence and change; and specific considerations regarding the formation and solution of human problems.

Chapter 4 discusses the techniques applied throughout the treatment, and explains the main procedures (strategies, tactics, techniques) employed. This discourse does not consist merely of descriptions of the course of therapy and strategies but goes on to show their efficacy in altering people's perceptions, behavior, and opinions. Examples of research and experiments are included, as well as references to comparable problems encountered in other scientific contexts. The therapy process is presented systematically in a detailed format that shows the precise therapeutic aims of each one and the specific strategies used to achieve those aims. The cases demonstrate the efficacy of these methods and show how therapy can be a swift, well-planned journey whose point of departure, direction, destination, and length can be fairly clear from the beginning.

Chapter 5 presents advanced techniques for treating specific pathologies as determined by long-term experimental-empirical research. This rigorous work is one of Nardone's most important and creative contributions to the evolution of brief therapy.

Chapter 6 presents some interesting and unusual case histories. They demonstrate why, when seeking a solution to specific human problems, the therapist needs to combine a knowledge of systematic strategies and techniques with inventiveness and mental versatility. This is necessary because in order to find new, effective solutions to a problem, occasionally we must deviate from traditional conceptual schemes, from our usual ways of perceiving and reacting to our clients. Both knowledge and flexibility are essential for the rapid substitution of any ineffective solutions hitherto attempted.

Chapter 7 concludes the book on a note that is rare in our work—namely, a systematic, thorough evaluation of the results obtained by the application of this technique to a large and varied group of subjects over a ten-year period. The outcomes prove that this approach is definitely efficacious; it can solve the problems to which it is applied; and results are obtained in a matter of weeks or months, as opposed to the years normally required by traditional psychotherapy.

I believe this book to be of fundamental importance for all professionals interested in brief psychotherapy based on systemic, Ericksonian concepts. I recommend it to all those who are interested in the formation and solution of human problems because, although essentially professional in nature, it is readable and comprehensible, and the strategies described may be applied not only to psychotherapy but also to more general, nonclinical interpersonal situations.

Paul Watzlawick
Palo Alto, California

1

IF YOU DESIRE TO SEE, LEARN HOW TO ACT

The title of this chapter is borrowed from an essay by the famous cybernetician Heinz von Foerster. He calls it his aesthetic imperative. Although postulated in a different context (Foerster 1984), it nevertheless expresses what I consider to be an important aspect of the evolution of therapy. (The omission of the prefix *psycho-* before the word *therapy* is no slip, which I explain in the course of my presentation.) I do not know exactly how the inverse of von Foerster's imperative—the idea that in order to act differently, one must first learn to see the world differently—arose and acquired dogmatic dominance in our field. For as different and even as contradictory as the classic schools and philosophies of psychotherapy are among themselves, one of the assumptions they firmly share is that the understanding of the origin and the evolution of a problem in the

This chapter is a revision of Chapter 1 of the book *The Art of Change*, Jossey-Bass Publishers, San Francisco, 1993.

past is the precondition for its solution in the present. Undoubtedly, one compelling reason for this perspective is that it is embedded in the model of linear scientific thought and inquiry, a model that must be credited with the vertiginous progress of science during the last three hundred years.

Until the middle of the twentieth century, relatively few people questioned the supposedly final validity of a scientific worldview based on strictly deterministic, linear causality. Freud, for instance, saw no reason to doubt it. "At least in the older and more mature sciences, there is even today a solid ground-work which is only modified and improved, but no longer demolished" (Freud 1933, p. 58). This statement is of more than historic interest. Seen from the vantage point of the present time, it makes us aware of the evanescence of scientific paradigms whether we have read Kuhn (1970) or not.

One would naively believe that the history of the twentieth century alone should leave no doubt about the horrifying consequences produced by the illusion of having found the ultimate truth and, therefore, the "final solution." But the evolution of our field—since it usually is thirty years in arrears—has not quite arrived at this realization. Endless hours of "scientific" debates and tens of thousands of pages in books and scientific journals are still wasted in order to show that since "my way" of seeing reality is the right and true one, anybody who sees it differently is necessarily wrong. A good example of this fallacy is Edward Glover's (1956) book on Freud and Jung, in which this eminent author employs approximately two hundred pages to say what could be said in one sentence, namely, that Jung was wrong because he did not agree with Freud. This, incidentally, is what Glover finally says himself on page 190: "As we have seen, the most consistent trend of Jungian psychology is its negation of every important aspect of Freudian theory."

Clearly, to write such a book would have to be considered a waste of time unless the author and his readers are convinced that their view is right and any other view therefore is wrong.

There is something else that our professional evolution no longer lets us disregard. The dogmatic assumption that the discovery of the real causes of the present problem constitutes a *conditio sine qua non* (essential condition) for change creates what the philosopher Karl Popper has called a self-sealing proposition, that is, a hypothesis that is validated both by its success and its failure and thus one that becomes unfalsifiable. In practical terms, if a patient improves as a result of what in classical theory is called insight, this obviously proves the correctness of the hypothesis about the need to lift forgotten, repressed causes into consciousness. If the patient does not improve, this proves that the search for these causes has not yet proceeded deep enough into the past. The hypothesis wins either way.

A related consequence of the belief in possessing the ultimate truth is the ease with which the believer can dismiss any evidence to the contrary. The mechanism involved here is well known to philosophers of science, but usually not to clinicians. A good example is the review of a book dealing with the behavior therapy of phobias. It culminates in the reviewer's statement that the author defines phobias "in a way that is acceptable only to conditioning theorists and does not fulfill the criteria of the psychiatric definition of this disorder. Therefore, his statements should not apply to phobias, but to some other condition" (Salzman 1968, p. 476). The conclusion is inescapable: a phobia that improves in response to behavior therapy is for this reason no phobia. One gets the impression that it sometimes seems more important to save the theory than the patient, and one is reminded of Hegel's dictum that if the facts don't comply with the theory, so much the worse for the facts.

(Hegel was probably far too great a mind to have meant this in any other than a facetious sense. But I may be wrong. Hegelian Marxism certainly means it dead seriously—and, again, the word *dead* is not to be taken as a mere slip of the tongue.)

Finally, we can no longer afford to remain blind to yet another epistemological error, as Gregory Bateson might have called it. Only too often we find that the limitations inherent in a given hypothesis are attributed to the phenomena that that hypothesis is supposed to elucidate. For instance, within the framework of psychodynamic theory, symptom removal must necessarily lead to symptom substitution and exacerbation, not because this complication is in some sense inherent in the nature of the human mind but because it imposes itself logically and necessarily from the premises of that theory.

In the midst of such complicated thoughts, don't we all occasionally have a disconcerting fantasy: If the little green men from Mars arrive and ask us to explain our techniques for effecting human change, and if we then told them, would they not scratch their heads (or their equivalent) in disbelief and ask us why we have arrived at such complicated, abstruse, and far-fetched theories, rather than first of all investigating how human change comes about naturally, spontaneously, and on an everyday basis? I, for one, would try to point out to them that there have been at least some historic forerunners of that eminently reasonable and practical idea that Heinz von Foerster so well summarized in his aesthetic imperative. One of them is Franz Alexander, to whom we owe the important concept of the corrective emotional experience. He explains:

> It is not necessary—nor is it possible—during the course of treatment to recall every feeling that has been repressed. Therapeutic results can be achieved without the patient's recalling all important details of his past history; indeed, good therapeutic results have come in

cases in which not a single forgotten memory has been brought to the surface. Ferenczi and Rank were among the first to recognize this principle and apply it to therapy. However, the early belief that the patient "suffers from memories" has so deeply penetrated the minds of the analysts that even today it is difficult for many to recognize that the patient is suffering not so much from his memories as from his incapacity to deal with his actual problems of the moment. The past events have of course prepared the way for his present difficulties, but then every person's reactions are dependent upon behavior patterns formed in the past. . . . This new corrective experience may be supplied by the transference relationship, by new experiences in life, or by both. [Alexander and French 1946, p. 22]

While Alexander attributes far greater importance to a patient's experiences in the transference situation (because these are not chance events, but are provided by the analyst's refusal to be forced into a parental role), he is quite aware also to what extent the outside world may provide just such random events as will effect profound and lasting change. In fact, Alexander (1956) mentions specifically that "such intensive revelatory emotional experiences give us the clue for those puzzling therapeutic results which are obtained in a considerably shorter time than usual in psychoanalysis" (p. 92). In this connection, Alexander (Alexander and French 1946) refers to Victor Hugo's (1862) Jean Valjean in *Les Misérables*, an imprisoned peasant who, upon his release from a long jail sentence that brutalized him even more, is caught stealing the bishopric's silver. He is brought before the bishop, but instead of calling him a thief, the bishop asks him very kindly why he left behind the two silver candlesticks that were also part of the bishop's gift to him. This kindness totally upsets Valjean's worldview. In the mental imbalance produced by the bishop's reframing of the situation, Valjean meets a little boy, Gervais, who is playing with his coins and drops a forty-sou piece. Valjean puts his foot on the coin and refuses to let Gervais have it back. The boy cries, desperately pleads for his money, and eventually runs away. Only then does it dawn on Valjean how hideously cruel his behavior—which only an hour earlier would have been a matter of course for him—now appears in light of the bishop's kindness toward him. He runs after Petit-Gervais but cannot find him. Hugo explains:

> He felt indistinctly that the priest's forgiveness was the most formidable assault by which he had been shaken; that his hardening would be permanent if he resisted this clemency; that if he yielded he must renounce that hatred with which the actions of other men had filled his soul during so many years, and which pleased him; that this time he must either conquer or be vanquished; and that the struggle, a colossal and final struggle, had begun between his wickedness and that man's goodness. [p. 95]

We must bear in mind that *Les Misérables* was written in 1862, half a century before the advent of psychoanalytic theory, and that it would be a bit preposterous to assume that the bishop was simply an early-day analyst. Rather, what Hugo shows is the timeless human experience of profound change arising out of another person's unexpected and unexpectable action.

I do not know whether another eminent psychiatrist and author, Michael Balint, has explicitly incorporated Franz Alexander's concept of the corrective emotional experience into his own work. However, in his book *The Basic Fault* (1968), he mentions the classic somersault incident, which provides an excellent illustration of such an experience. He was working with a patient, "an attractive, vivacious, rather flirtatious girl in her late twenties, whose main complaint was an inability to achieve anything" (p. 128) This was due, in part, to her "crippling fear of uncertainty whenever she had to take any risk, that is, make a decision" (p. 128). Balint describes how, after two years of psychoanalytic treatment,

> she was given the interpretation that apparently the most important thing for her was to keep her head safely up, with both feet firmly planted on the ground. In response, she mentioned that ever since her earliest childhood she could never do a somersault; although at various periods she tried desperately to do one. I then said: "What about it now?" whereupon she got up from the couch and, to her great amazement, did a perfect somersault without any difficulty. This proved to be a real breakthrough. Many changes followed, in her emotional, social, and professional life, all towards greater freedom and elasticity. Moreover, she managed to get permission to sit for, and passed, a most difficult postgraduate professional examination, became engaged, and was married. [pp. 128–129]

Balint then proceeds to use almost two pages to prove that this remarkable, immediate change was, after all, not in contradiction to object relations theory. "I wish to emphasize," he concludes, "that the satisfaction did not replace interpretation, it was in addition to it" (p. 134).

The first comprehensive shift in the evolution of our understanding of human change occurred in 1937, when Jean Piaget published his seminal work *La Construction du Réel Chez l'Enfant*, which became available in English in 1954 under the title *The Construction of Reality in the Child*. Here, Piaget proves, on the basis of painstaking observations, that the child *constructs* his reality by exploratory actions, rather than by first forming an image of the world through his perceptions and then beginning to act accordingly. Only a few passages from his enormously detailed study can be quoted here to support this contention. In what Piaget calls the third stage of the development of object concepts, between 3 and 6 months of age, "the child begins to grasp what he sees, to bring before his eyes the objects he touches, in short to coordinate his visual universe with the tactile universe" (Piaget 1937, p. 13). Later, in the same chapter, Piaget states that these actions lead to a greater degree of assumed object permanence, which

> is attributed to vanished images, since the child expects to find them again not only in the very place where they were left but also in places within the extension of their trajectory (reaction to falling, interrupted prehension, etc.). But in comparing this stage with the following ones we prove that this permanence remains exclusively connected with the action in progress and does not yet imply the idea of substantial permanence independent of the organism's sphere of activity. All that the child assumes is that in continuing to turn his head or to lower it he will see a certain image which has just disappeared, that in lowering his hand he will again find the tactile impression experienced shortly before, etc. . . .
>
> In effect, at this stage the child does not know the mechanism of his own actions, and hence does not dissociate them from the things themselves; he knows only their total and undifferentiated schema (which we have called the schema of assimilation) comprising in a single act the data of external perception as well as the internal impressions that are effective and kinesthetic, etc., in nature. . . . The child's universe is still only a totality of pictures emerging from nothingness at the moment of the action, to return to nothingness at the moment when the action is finished. There is added to it only the circumstance that the images subsist no longer than before, because the child tries to make these actions last longer than in the past; in extending them either he rediscovers the vanished images or else he supposes them to be at his disposal in the very situation in which the act in progress began. [pp. 41–43]

The importance of Piaget's findings for our work can hardly be overstated. In the gradual unfolding of his research results, Piaget not only shows how the idea of a world "out there," independent of oneself, is the outcome of exploratory actions, but also explains the development of such basic concepts as causality, time, and eventually, as he calls it, "the elaboration of the universe." If this be so, then, obviously, different actions may lead to the construction of different "realities." However, before discussing this subject, some further milestones along the evolutionary path of therapy must be mentioned.

It may seem far-fetched, indeed, that in order to reach the next milestone I go back in time to Blaise Pascal, who, in his Pensée 223, developed an argument that has become known as Pascal's wager. It is of interest to us therapists because, although theological in form, it deals with a problem very close to home. Pascal examines the age-old question of how a nonbeliever can arrive, by and through himself, at a state of faith. His suggestion is intriguing: behave as if you already believed—for instance, by praying, using holy water, partaking in the sacraments, and so forth. Out of these actions, faith will follow. And since there is at least a probability that God exists, to say nothing of the potential benefits (peace of mind and final salvation), your stakes in this game are small. "*Qu'avez-vous à perdre* (What do you have to lose)?" he asks rhetorically.

Pascal's wager gave rise to innumerable arguments, speculations, and treatises. Let me mention just one of them. In his fascinating book *Ulysses and the Sirens*, the Norwegian philosopher Jon Elster (1979) takes up Pascal's thought and goes on to show that one cannot decide to believe something without the necessity to forget the decision:

The implication of this argument is that the decision to believe can only be carried out successfully if accompanied by a decision to forget, viz., a decision to forget the decision to believe. This, however, is just as paradoxical as the decision to believe. . . . The most efficient procedure would be to start up a single causal process with the double effect of inducing belief and making you forget that it was ever started up. Asking to be hypnotized is one such mechanism. [p. 50]

This seems crucial to my subject. To forget on purpose is one thing, and it is impossible. But to do something because the reason, impulse, or suggestion for this action comes from the outside, as the result of either a chance event or a deliberate action or suggestion by someone else—in other words, in communicative interaction with another person—is quite another thing.

At this point I have to take up the evolution of modern family therapy, which no longer asks, Why is the identified patient behaving in this bizarre, irrational fashion? but rather, In what sort of human system does this behavior make sense and is it perhaps the only possible behavior? and, What sort of solutions has this system so far attempted? But these considerations would make my discussion overly lengthy. Let me merely point out that at this juncture therapy has little, if anything, to do with concepts beginning with the prefix *psycho-*, such as psychology, psychopathology, and psychotherapy. For it is no longer just the individual, monadic psyche that concerns us here, but the superindividual structures arising out of the interactions between individuals (Watzlawick 1985).

The vast majority of the problems we want to change are related not to the properties of objects or of situations—to the reality of the first order (Watzlawick 1976)—but to the meaning, the sense, and the value that we have come to attribute to these objects or situations (their second-order reality). "It is not the things them-selves that worry us, but the opinions that we have about those things," said Epictetus some 1,900 years ago. And most of us know the answer to the question about the difference between an opti-mist and a pessimist: the optimist says of a bottle of wine that it is half full; the pessimist says that it is half empty. This is the same reality of the first order—a bottle with some wine in it—but two very different second-order realities, resulting, in fact, in two different worlds. Seen in this way, one may say that all therapy is concerned with bringing about changes in the way people have constructed their second-order realities (which they are totally convinced are the real reality).

In traditional psychotherapy one attempts to achieve this through the use of indicative language, or description, explanation, confron-tation, interpretation, and so forth. This is the language of classical science and of linear causality. However, it does not lend itself very well to the description of nonlinear, systemic phenomena (for ex-ample, human relationships), and it lends itself even less to the com-munication of new experiences and realizations for which the past provides no understanding and that lie outside a given person's re-ality construction.

But what other language is there? The answer is given, for instance, by George Spencer Brown (1973) in his book *Laws of Form*, where, almost as an aside, he defines the concept of injunctive lan-guage. Taking mathematical communication as his point of depar-ture, he writes:

> It may be helpful at this stage to realize that the primary form of mathematical communication is not description, but injunction. In this respect it is comparable with practical art forms, like cookery, in which the taste of a cake, although literally indescribable, can be

conveyed to a reader in the form of a set of injunctions called a recipe. Music is a similar art form. The composer does not even attempt to describe the set of sounds he has in mind, much less the set of feelings occasioned through them, but writes down a set of commands which, if they are obeyed by the reader, can result in a reproduction, to the reader, of the composer's original experience. [p. 77]

Brown also comments on the role of injunctive language in the training of scientists:

Even natural science appears to be more dependent upon injunction than we are usually prepared to admit. The professional initiation of the man of science consists not so much in reading the proper textbooks as in obeying injunctions such as "look down that microscope." But it is not out of order for men of science, having looked down the microscope, now to describe to each other, and to discuss amongst themselves, what they have seen, and to write papers and textbooks describing it. [p. 78]

In other words, if we manage to get clients to undertake actions that in and by themselves were always possible, but that the clients did not perform because in their second-order reality there was no sense or reason to carry them out, then through the very performance of these actions the clients will experience something that no amount of explaining and interpreting may ever have revealed or made attainable. And with this we have arrived at Heinz von Foerster's imperative: if you desire to see, learn how to act.

Needless to say, people may strenuously resist the request to perform such actions. The classical example is Galileo Galilei's contemporaries who disdained to look through his telescope because they knew without looking that what he claimed to see could not be the case (within the limits of their second-order reality, that is, geocentricity). Remember, if the facts don't comply with the theory, so much the worse for the facts.

Milton Erickson's work introduces the concept of injunctive language. In the second half of his professional life, Erickson increasingly utilized direct behavior prescriptions outside trance states in order to achieve therapeutic change. Being a master in dealing with resistance, he gave us an important rule: learn and use the patient's language. This, too, is a radical departure from classical psychotherapy, where a great deal of time is spent in the beginning stages of treatment in the attempt to teach the patient a new "language," that is, the conceptualizations of the particular school of therapy that the therapist subscribes to. Only when patients have begun to think in terms of this epistemology, to see themselves, their problems, their lives, in this perspective, is therapeutic change attempted within this framework. Needless to say, this process may take a long time. In hypnotherapy the opposite takes place; it is the therapist who learns the patient's language and reality construction (as we would call it nowadays), and then gives suggestions in this language, thereby minimizing resistance (and time).

Outside its therapeutic applications, the study of injunctive language had its origins in the work of the Austrian philosopher Ernst Mally. In his book *Grundgesetze des Sollens* (1926), Mally developed a theory of wishes and commands that he called deontic logic.

Another important contribution to this subject can be found in the work of British philosopher of language John L. Austin (1962). In his famous Harvard Lectures in 1955, he identified a particular form of communication that he called performative speech acts or performative sentences. "The term performative will be used in a variety of cognate ways and constructions, much as the term imperative is. The name is derived, of course, from perform, the usual verb with the noun action. It indicates that the issuing of the utterance is the performing of an action—it is not normally thought of as just saying something" (p. 6).

For instance, if I say, "He promises to return the book tomorrow," I describe (in indicative language) an action, a speech act, by that person. But if I say, "I promise to return the book tomorrow," saying "I promise" is itself the promise, the action. In Austin's terminology, the first example (the description) is called a constative, while the second is a performative speech act. In Lecture IV, Austin points to the difference between the statements "I am running" and "I apologize." The former is a mere report of an action; the latter is itself the action, is the apology. Other examples from everyday life are "I take this woman to be my lawful wedded wife," "I name this ship Queen Elizabeth," "I give and bequeath my watch to my brother." In all of these and in countless analogous speech acts, a concrete result is achieved, while my saying "winter is coming" does not make the winter come. Of course, a number of preconditions have to be met for a performative speech act to obtain or be effective. For instance, past disappointment or lies may make me doubt the promise; the apology must not be offered in a sneering, sarcastic tone of voice; the ceremony of naming a ship has to be an established procedure in a given culture. But if and when these preconditions are met, a reality is created by the performative utterance, and whoever subsequently referred to that ship as the Joseph Stalin would be considered somewhat deranged.

I have barely scratched the surface of Austin's work in this specialized area of linguistics, that is, his ideas on "how to do things with words." But I hope that even these brief references will reveal some of the richness and the relevance of it for our work.

Of a particularly mind-boggling effect are the so-called self-fulfilling prophecies, known to unorthodox therapists and stockbrokers alike, but not to weather forecasters: imagined effect produces concrete cause; the future (not the past) determines the present; the prophecy of the event leads to the event of the prophecy (Watzlawick 1984).

I am convinced that injunctive language will acquire a central place within the frame of modern therapeutic techniques. It has always occupied this place in hypnotherapy. For what is a hypnotic suggestion if not an injunction to behave as if something were the case—something that does become the case (that is, becomes "real") as a result of having been carried out? But this is tantamount to saying that injunctions can construct realities, just as chance events can have this effect not only in human lives, but also in cosmic as well as biological evolution. In this connection, it would be tempting to go off on a tangent, into questions of self-organization, or what Prigogine (1980) called *dissipative structures*—a subject that would exceed the limits of my competence and my time.

Why is there a crucial difference between something originating within myself and an impulse that comes from the outside? Several answers offer themselves, but none seems convincing. That it is so is no secret. In our own lives we have little difficulty creating the same disaster as our so-called patients do in their lives, and to tickle oneself is never as ticklish as being tickled by somebody else. However, to go back to Pascal, his behavior prescription is to behave *as if* you already believed, which clearly points to the initially quite fictional nature of this class of interventions. And it is this fictionality that creates doubts. The common objection is that even if they are successful, their effect cannot last. After all, they are only make believe, an as-if fiction. Sooner or later, probably sooner, they must run up against the hard facts of reality and be defeated.

Here is the counterargument: The idea of introducing an as-if assumption into a situation and thereby arriving at concrete results is by no means a recent one. It goes back at least to the year

1911, when the German philosopher Hans Vaihinger published his *Philosophie des Als Ob*, whose English title is *The Philosophy of "As If"* (1924). If it were not for the fact that Alfred Adler (and, to a lesser degree, also Freud) had already recognized the importance of these ideas, their application to our field could very well be called the therapy of as if, or the therapy of "planned chance events." Vaihinger presents an astounding richness of examples, drawn from all branches of science as well as from everyday life, showing that we always work with unproven and unprovable assumptions that nevertheless lead to concrete, practical results. There is no proof that man is endowed with free will and is therefore responsible for his actions. However, I know of no society, culture, or civilization, past or present, in which people did not behave as if this were the case, because without this fictitious assumption, practical, concrete social order would be impossible. The idea of the square root of minus one is totally fictional. It is not only intellectually unimaginable, it also violates the basic rules of arithmetic; yet, mathematicians, physicists, engineers, computer programmers, and others have nonchalantly included this fiction in their equations and have arrived at very concrete results—such as modern electronics.

The rules and patterns of interaction that a family or systems therapist claims to observe are quite obviously read into the observed phenomena by the therapist. They are not really there. And yet, to conduct therapy as if these patterns existed can lead to practical and quick results. Thus, the question is no longer, Which school of therapy is right? but rather, Which as-if assumptions produce better concrete results? Maybe the decline of dogma is approaching.

This way of conceptualizing and of trying to resolve human problems is gaining increasing attention as the traditional techniques of problem resolution seem to be reaching the limits of their usefulness. We are beginning to apply these methods to what may be called the specific pathologies of large systems. It does not seem totally utopian to imagine their application even to some of the most pressing and threatening problems of our planet, such as the maintenance of peace or the preservation of our biosphere. However, these attempts are too often beset by the same basic mistake that plays havoc in clinical work, namely, the assumption that since the problems are of enormous proportion, only some equally enormous, transcending solution has any chance of succeeding. The opposite appears to be the case. If we look at the history of the last few centuries, beginning with the French Revolution or even with the Inquisition, we see that invariably and without exception the worst atrocities were the direct result of grandiose and utopian attempts at improving the world. What the philosopher Karl Popper calls "a policy of small steps" is unacceptable to idealists and ideologists. Remember the aphorism that Gregory Bateson often mentioned: "He who would do good must do so in minute particulars. The general good is the plea of patriots, politicians, and knaves."

To convince ourselves, we only have to look at nature. Great changes are always catastrophic and cataclysmic. Negentropy—or anotropy, as George Vassiliou in Athens prefers to call it, in order to avoid the double negative—works patiently, silently, in small steps; yet it is the force behind evolution, self-organization, and higher complexity in the universe. I think that if we, as therapists, begin to see ourselves as the servants of negentropy, we will fulfill our function better than we do as supposed world-improvers and gurus. Heinz von Foerster (1984) defined this function in his ethical imperative: act always so as to increase the number of choices.

Many centuries ago this same outlook was expressed in a charming story:

After his death, the Sufi Abu Bakr Shibli appeared to one of his friends in a dream. "How has God treated you?" the friend asked. And the Sufi answered, "As I stood before His throne, He asked me, 'Do you know why I am forgiving you?' And I said, 'Because of my good deeds?' And God said, 'No, not because of those.' I asked, 'Because I was sincere in my adoration?' And God said, 'No.' I then said, 'Because of my pilgrimages and my journeys to acquire knowledge and to enlighten others?' And God again replied, 'No, not because of all this.' So I asked Him, 'Oh Lord, why then have you forgiven me?' And He answered, 'Do you remember how on a bitterly cold winter day you were walking through the streets of Baghdad and you saw a hungry kitten desperately trying to find shelter from the icy wind, and you had pity on it and picked it up and put it inside your fur and took it into your home?' I said, 'Yes, my Lord, I remember.' And God said, 'Because you were kind to that cat, Abu Bakr, because of that I have forgiven you.'" [Schimmel 1983, p. 16]

2

NONORDINARY LOGIC
FOR STRATEGIC
PROBLEM SOLVING

There is a serious aspect to stupidity which might, if
better directed, multiply the number of masterpieces.

E. M. Cioran, *Syllogisms of Bitterness*

FROM EPISTEMOLOGY TO LOGIC:
FOR BETTER GUIDELINES
IN BRIEF THERAPY

The field of applied psychotherapy often reveals some strange situations, among them an excessive number of complicated theories and a scarcity of practical contributions. This, in my opinion, is due to the fact that psychologists, psychiatrists, and psychotherapists usually ignore the logical and epistemological criteria that constitute the foundations of scientific knowledge.

Being either too theoretical or too reductive, they divide our discipline into general theoretical systems and clinical practice, often disregarding an instrument that has, since antiquity, guided thinkers in bringing together theory and practice—namely, logic. We therefore find a wide gap between the increasingly complex and often complicated formulations of the current epistemological debate on human mind, behavior, and change, and the frequently naive practical instructions for therapists.

Logic has always guided the planning of strategies and behavior. From ancient times to our days, logic has evolved as a very special field of research, normally reserved for mathematicians and philosophers, but also as an indispensable instrument for anyone who wishes to construct systematic projects for the solution of specific problems. We all consciously or unconsciously apply logic, from our most simple actions to our most complicated interactions, because logic is always at the basis of our planning of action sequences aimed toward an objective.

Psychotherapists, who are commonly thought to be very pragmatic technical specialists, have strangely forgotten or, worse, disregarded this field of theoretical and applied science. Consequently, "reductionism-determinism" and "complicationalism" are the only two basic types of logic found in psychotherapy.

The former type can be observed in models based on rigidly deterministic theories, such as psychoanalysis and behaviorism. Although on opposite sides, these two schools and their derivations share the same epistemology, based on a mechanistic and positivistic logical model. They follow Aristotelian, rationalistic, traditional principles based on concepts such as "scientific objectivity," "coherence," and the "principle of noncontradiction." Their rigid application of hypothetical and deductive logic where hypotheses and deductive processes are founded on an a priori deterministic theory has a strongly reductive effect on knowledge of mind and behavior.

This situation has produced a self-referential system, where the logic that guides clinical practice is rigidly determined by the same theoretical system that the logic itself is supposed to verify. In the virtual circle thus created, hypotheses are confirmed based on an unverified theory, and the theory is confirmed based on logical deductions construed by the same theory. This is essentially a form of causal circularity in which "unproved truths" verify each other.

The theorists whom I have called "complicationists," who are currently very much in vogue, are complicating the study of the human mind and behavior with their interpretations of the recent theory of complexity (Morin 1985) and constructivism. The seemingly more and more rigorous and articulate theories that they construct still remain unproved; they are lost within the complexity of their theories, and have forfeited any ability to plan effective and pragmatic intervention strategies. In this case, pure epistemology predominates to the detriment of the logic of intervention, due to the theorists' inability to move from the purely theoretical level to the structuring of clinical operations. I believe that this is due to the fact that, in recent years, many authors have placed too much emphasis on the epistemological aspects of psychotherapy, neglecting to give due attention to the evolution of disciplines that study the interaction of theories and practices in the construction and verification of models of intervention.

Modern logic offers some very interesting formulations that enable psychotherapists to take into account the complexity of human mind and behavior, as well as the need to construct efficient and effective strategies for reaching an objective. Significantly, this discipline, which has always concerned itself with problem solving, includes a branch called "strategic logic."

Strategic logic makes it possible to:

1. construct rigorous models on the basis of objectives, rather than on the dictates of some theory that prescribes the criteria for health and pathology, a priori;
2. use constitutive-deductive logic instead of hypothetical-deductive logic in the formation of strategies, thus ensuring that the solution will fit the problem, instead of forcing the problem to fit a solution derived from the hypotheses of normative and prescriptive theories;
3. have an ongoing self-corrective process, based on the observed effects, during the interaction between the solution and the problem, rather than persevering with solutions that do not produce positive effects, or that even (as is often the case) exacerbate the problem that they are supposed to solve, for no other reason than that these unsuccessful solutions are consistent and congruent with the chosen model of theory and practice.

The past decades have seen the development of new models of "paraconsistent" and non-alethic logic (Da Costa 1989a,b, Grana 1990) that lead us beyond the traditional Aristotelian logic of true or false and the principle of noncontradiction. These models make it possible to use interventions based on contradiction, paradox, and self-deception in a rigorous manner.

Unfortunately, as I have described above, traditional logic still underlies most formulations of psychotherapy, including those of the "complicationists" who use modern epistemology. I believe that by failing to consider that the use of logic is inevitable when moving from theory to practice, these theorists do not update their logical models and, thus, unconsciously introduce traditional logic in their modern epistemology.

For example, cognitive psychotherapy, which is one of the most innovative formulations in our field, presents the situation described above. The cognitive theory and epistemology are truly modern, but if we analyze their models of application, we discover that the Aristotelian logical principles of coherence and noncontradiction are still widely used.

For instance, the logic that guides the therapeutic intervention in cognitive psychotherapy aims to solve the contradictions within an individual's cognitive and emotional constructs, in order to develop internal consistency, as if an absence of internal contradictions in the individual's cognitive structure were equivalent to an absence of real psychological problems. This is a strictly rationalistic logical procedure, based on a hypothetical–deductive process that applies the principles of coherence and noncontradiction as an unquestionable base for the therapeutic objective, without considering that those principles were made obsolete about thirty years ago by the disciplines that study human interactions and their related logical processes. It is very strange to see a model based on constructivist theory become so reductive at the level of practical logic.

On the other hand, the theorists of psychotherapy often confuse the logical level of analyzing a phenomenon with that of constituting a model of intervention; in other words, they confuse epistemology with the construction of clinical models. This occurs in approaches that adopt the constructivistic theorctical perspective not just at the epistemological level, but as if it were a logic of intervention, thus suffering shipwreck within their own conceptual relativity.

As von Glasersfeld (1995), the greatest theorist of radical constructivism, clearly states, it should not surprise us that a problem solver sees the problematic experiential situation that he is working on as real. His task is technical, based on specific, circumscribed fields of experience, and his ability to solve the problem is not increased by epistemological considerations. Only when he has resolved the problem will he be able to adopt a philosophical attitude as a tool for the organization and understanding of the experience, rather than as a representation of reality.

In other words, the passage from the logical level of epistemology to that of practice requires an intermediate level represented by logic, that is, the method for forming specific models of intervention, as, indeed, happens in all applied sciences. In physics, for example, the theory of relativity or the principle of indetermination does not make physicists incapable of planning experimental protocols for specific projects, since, as von Glasersfeld points out, they consider the specific portion of reality that is the subject of their intervention as if it were true. Only after having obtained the results of their experiment can they adopt it as a tool for knowledge. In other words, we know a problem by its solution (Nardone 1996). This operative knowledge can then be used both at the logical level of epistemology and at the logical level of structuring strategies for intervention.

To avoid falling into the naive forms of logical and methodological error described above, those of us who are involved in planning models of clinical intervention must keep separate the logical levels of:

1. Theory-epistemology (cognitive-theoretical level)
2. The strategy or model (cognitive-operative level)
3. The single therapeutic maneuver or technique (operative-cognitive level).

A different perspective is called for, according to the level of logic that we are dealing with. At level 1, we must adopt a cognitive-theoretical perspective; at level 2 a cognitive-operative perspective; and at level 3 an operative-cognitive perspective. This enables us to work both creatively and systematically, making fruitful use of the contributions of empirical experience as the basis for a structure of intervention that is capable of prediction, and is constituted according to advanced logical and epistemological criteria, in a constant circle of retroactions between the operative and the cognitive perspective (Salvini 1995), a circle that guards against self-sealing rigidities (Popper 1972, 1973) and keeps the model in a constant self-corrective evolution.

NONORDINARY LOGIC
AND BRIEF THERAPY

By using strategic and paraconsistent logic we can, as we have already mentioned, make rigorous use of nonordinary logical procedures in a therapeutic context. These procedures enable us to construct stratagems that can break pathogenic balances of perception and reaction, which are usually resistant to changes induced through ordinary logic. In other words, in cases where ordinary logical procedures (based on the revelations and knowledge of the formation and persistence of the problem with consequent instructions as to how to proceed in order to change) fail, we may turn to alternative logical procedures, appropriate for phenomena that persist on the basis of nonordinary types of logic. In our view, this applies to most nonlinear phenomena connected with the interactions between the subject and reality, and particularly to cases in which this interaction has led to pathological mental and behavioral expressions.

A few concrete examples may be useful in clarifying this concept. If we attempt to use reason in convincing an obsessive-compulsive patient to stop his pathological rituals, we will obtain no effect. Instead, we use a stratagem based on the logic of paradox and belief, as in the following prescription: "Every time you enact one of your rituals, you must repeat it five times—exactly five times, no more, no less. You can avoid doing it at all, but if you do it once, you must do it no more and no less than five times."* The usual effect is that the patient quickly stops the rituals.

This prescription employs the same logic as that which underlies the persistence of the pathology, but changes its direction: the force of the symptom is turned against the disorder, with the effect of breaking its perverse balance. The injunction to "ritually" repeat the rituals leads the person to construct a different reality from the reality characterized by uncontrollable compulsions. Within this new reality, the person sees the possibility of not performing any rituals, since the ritual is not uncontrollably spontaneous here, but prescribed and voluntary. We take control of the symptom by constructing another structurally similar symptom that cancels the former. But since the latter is a deliberate construction, it can be deliberately refused, as in the ancient Chinese stratagem of "making the enemy go into the attic, and then removing the ladder."

With patients who suffer from agoraphobia, we can make rational arguments for years on end without ever convincing them to go out alone. Instead, by using a logic of self-deception and belief, we can give this injunctive prescription:

---

* This prescription, like the others that follow, is a technique that has been formalized in the treatment protocols for phobic and obsessive symptoms (Nardone 1996, Nardone and Watzlawick 1993).

You are now going to do something very important. Go to the door and do a pirouette. Open the door, go out and do another pirouette. Then go down the stairs; when you get to the main door, do one pirouette before and one after stepping out of the building. Turn left and keep walking, doing a pirouette every fifty steps, until you get to a fruit store. Do a pirouette before entering the store; then buy the largest and ripest apple you can find. Then walk back here, doing a pirouette every fifty steps, one before entering the building and one after. I will be waiting for you here.

We usually obtain both the apple and the patient's first important corrective emotional experience.

In this case, the logic behind the intervention is to construct a suggestive, ritualized sequence of seemingly illogical actions that move the person's attention away from the fear, and onto the accomplishment of the task. We prescribe this task as if it were a kind of magic. Thus, we have the added effect of self-deception, "sailing the sea without the sky's knowledge," and enchanted belief, as if making pirouettes could really scare the fears away. In other words, we have an invented reality that produces concrete effects.

A prescription with a less complex logical and linguistic structure, which is therefore more easily applied by therapists without a high degree of rhetorical ability (which is, on the contrary, indispensable for applying the maneuvers described above) is the "as if" prescription (Nardone and Watzlawick 1993). Because it is simple and flexible, the "as if" prescription can be applied to a wide range of problems. For example, we might say to a person who suffers from persecution manias and believes that everyone hates him or, at the very least, rejects him: "I would like you to think about how you would behave differently, as if you were convinced that you were very likable, and that everyone thought you desirable and wanted to be with you. Choose one of the things that comes to mind, and apply it. Every day, do something small but concrete, as if that's how you felt. It's an experiment. Try it."

As the reader can easily imagine, small but concrete actions of this kind usually overturn the habitual interaction between this patient and his reality. In those moments when he adopts a different attitude toward other people, other people will adopt a different attitude toward him, and he will thus have the experience of feeling liked and wanted. As both logicians and social scientists know, prophetic beliefs are self-fulfilling.

To explain this technique more clearly, suppose the patient enters a café thinking that he is disliked and unwanted. Let us try to put ourselves in the place of the others who are in the café and see this person coming in and looking around suspiciously. What will they do? Obviously, they will look back at him suspiciously. Thus, the final effect is that his supposition that he is disliked and unwanted will be confirmed, without his realizing that all this is a self-made construction of reality.

If the person manages to change the attitude that has led to this dysfunctional reality construction even just once a day, in some apparently insignificant situation, he will provoke a concrete corrective emotional experience that can easily be increased by increasing his "as if" actions and attitudes, until a new, functional reality is constructed and has replaced the previous one.

All this occurs based on an induced self-deception, which changes the direction of the believed prophecy, completely overturning the effect of the prophecy on the person's experience, and gradually leading to a change in the person's beliefs and perceptions of reality.

As we will describe in detail in the following chapters, the planning of specific interventions for particular forms of problems has been the main object of our research at the Arezzo Brief Strategic Therapy Center for the past decade; we might therefore cite many other equally creative and logically rigorous examples. What all these maneuvers have in common is the use of nonordinary logical mechanisms such as the logic of self-deception, paradox, belief, and contradiction. The type of logic is selected on the basis of the characteristics of the problem and the objective to be reached.

Thus, the construction of even a single prescription or reframing is planned on the basis of strategic logic. The planning of interventions is guided by the objective in front of us, not by the theory behind us, which is in need of confirmation.

For some maneuvers to be carried out by the patients and be effective, therapists must use suggestion and persuasion in their communication. This fundamentally important subject is discussed at length in Chapter 5.

The use of modern paraconsistent strategic logic enables us not only to use logical tactics and stratagems as single maneuvers for loosening up certain pathological blocks at the operative-cognitive level, but also to organize the problem-solving process in precise sequences from the very beginning of the intervention, that is, at the cognitive-operative level. This passage makes it possible to construct models of intervention that are specifically suited for particular types of problems (Nardone 1996, Nardone and Verbitz 1999) and therefore are not only more effective, but also capable of anticipating the possible developments of the therapeutic interaction.

The therapy thus becomes a process of strategic problem solving where, like in a chess game, the experienced player always keeps in mind which strategy will lead to checkmate as he responds to the adversary's moves. In other words, we try to predict the possible reactions to each single maneuver, and plan possible tactical or technical variations to the initial strategy on the basis of the observed effects, with the aim of reaching checkmate, which in therapy is the joint victory of the therapist and the patient over the problem at hand, as soon as possible.

However, the leap in logical level must never be considered conclusive. As in the chess game, there are infinite possible combinations. Moreover, the interaction between the operative-cognitive level and the cognitive-operative level of logic produces those important clinical innovations that make possible the simultaneously rigorous and creative evolution of a model for the solution of human problems.

This logic model underlying the advanced model of brief strategic therapy is often called too simplistic by its detractors. It is not simplistic at all. Although the techniques of brief strategic therapy may seem simple, they are based on a complex and well-constructed epistemology and logic of intervention. In contrast, some apparently complex interventions turn out to be based on truly reductive logical and epistemological models. We should be careful not to confuse complications with complexity. We also need to keep in mind that while it is easy to perform complex tasks in a complicated manner, it is difficult to make complicated things simple, and even more difficult to find simple solutions to complex problems; for this, a measure of genius is often required.

3

HERESIES OF THE STRATEGIC APPROACH

The true mystery of the world is the visible, not the invisible.

Oscar Wilde, *The Picture of Dorian Gray*

Chapters 1 and 2 have pointed out the direct conflict among traditional concepts of psychotherapy. One who holds the theoretical perspective presented here is a true "heretic" in terms of classical psychotherapeutic theory and practice. The strategic approach to the treatment of psychic disturbances and behaviors is indeed heretical with respect to the majority of psychotherapeutic models. Consequently, before beginning a detailed exposition, it is important to chart the major points of difference between the strategic approach and the orthodox theories of psychotherapy.

CHOOSE PROBABILITY OVER "TRUTH"

To know the truth one must imagine myriads of falsehoods. For what is truth? In matters of religion, it is simply the opinion that has survived. In matters of science, it is the ultimate sensation. In matters of art, it is one's last mood.

Oscar Wilde, *The Artist as Critic*

The therapist who adopts the strategic approach to human problems can appropriately be considered a psychotherapeutic heretic (in the etymological sense of the term, as "one who has the capacity of choice"), insofar as he or she does not become entrapped either in a rigid interpretive model of human nature or in a stiffly orthodox psychological and psychiatric paradigm. The strategic approach to therapy, linked directly to the contemporary philosophy of constructivist knowledge (Elster 1979, 1985, Glasersfeld 1979, 1984, 1995, Foerster 1970, 1974a, 1981, 1984, Mahoney 1991, Maturana 1978, Nardone 1991, 1993, 1996, Piaget 1970, 1971, Stolzenberg 1978, Varela 1975, 1979, Watzlawick 1976, 1984) is based on the assertion of the impossibility—on the part of any science—of offering an absolutely true and definitive explanation of reality. There is not only one reality but many realities, determined by the perspective of the observer and by the instruments used for observation. From this epistemological perspective, every interpretive model that presupposes an absolutely true and final explanation of nature and of human behavior is refuted because every model of this type falls inevitably into the trap of self-referentiality (a sort of naming itself, or self-justification). In the words of the epistemologist Popper, no theory can find its confirmation within itself or through the means of its own instruments without avoiding its "nonfalsifiability."* Popper also expresses succinctly—with the definition of self-sealing theories or propositions—the phenomenon relative to those theoretical models that protect themselves from falsification: closed all-encompassing systems, in which one finds the explanation for everything. But precisely because of this characteristic, such theories take on the role of "religious" conceptions and are thus not models of scientific knowledge. For Bateson (1979), science is a mode of perception, of organizing and giving significance to observations, thereby constructing subjective theories whose value is not definitive.

For the clinician, theories must not be irrefutable truths, but hypotheses related to the world, partial points of view, useful for describing and organizing observable data so as to achieve successful therapies or to correct unsuccessful ones. Accordingly, it is useful to recall that

it is precisely from the psychologists dedicated to the study of how we know that the notion comes that human beings, insofar as they are "thinking organisms," do not operate directly on the reality that they encounter but on the perceptive transformations which

---

* Since 1931, when Gödel published his famous undecidability theorem using *Principia Mathematica* as his basis (Whitehead and Russell 1910–1913), we have safely been able to abandon the hope that any system complex enough to include arithmetic (or, as Tarski has shown, any language of that complexity) will ever be able to prove its consistency within its own framework. This proof can only come from the outside, based on additional axioms, premises, concepts, comparisons, and the like, which the original system itself cannot generate or prove, and which are themselves again only provable by recourse to a yet wider framework, and so on in an infinite regress of metasystems, metametasystems, and so forth. In keeping with the basic postulates of *Principia Mathematica*, any statement about a collection (and the proof of the consistency is one such statement) involves all of the collection and cannot, must not, therefore, be part of it (Watzlawick et al. 1974).

form their experience of the world. Therefore, "categorizations," "schemes," "attributions," "inferences," "heuristics," and "conceptualizations" constitute the representational systems through which we can realize diverse configurations and explanations of the world. In the same way, for example, a telescope and a radio-telescope offer different representations of the same celestial bodies and their properties. [Salvini 1988, p. 7]

The strategic approach is not based on a theory that describes human nature in terms of the concepts of behavioral and mental health or normality in opposition to those of pathology, as is the case in traditional theories of psychotherapy. Instead, it is concerned with how humans cope with the problems of existence, with the interaction between individuals, and with the perceptions and relations individuals experience within themselves, with others, and with the world. It is not concerned with objects and subjects in and by themselves, but with the object/subject in relation, since we are convinced of the impossibility of extrapolating a subject from its interactive context. Recall a famous metaphor of Glasersfeld: when we encounter a locked door, what is of interest to us is not the lock in itself—its nature and intrinsic mechanism—but only the means of finding the key that will open it.

FIRST HERESY: PASSING FROM CLOSED TO OPEN THEORETICAL SYSTEMS

The focus of attention for the strategic therapist is the interdependent relations that each person experiences within self, with others, and with the world. The objective is their functioning, not in general and absolute terms of normality, but in terms of the entirely personal realities that vary from person to person, as well as from context to context. Therefore, the first heresy is the passing from closed to open theoretical systems, from the concept of scientific truth to that of probability; from deterministic linear causality to the more elastic circular causality; from orthodoxy to methodological doubt. In other words, one moves from the fideistic attitude of the believer to the skeptical perspective of the researcher, in the conviction that the fundamental criterion of validation and verification of a therapeutic model is not in its theoretical architecture or the profundity of its analyses, but in its heuristic value and its capacity for authentic intervention, measured in terms of its efficacy and effectiveness in the resolution of the problems to which it is applied. The strategies are devised on the basis of the objective to reach, and not, as usual for orthodox psychotherapies, on the basis of the theory to protect.

SECOND HERESY:
FOCUS ON HOW RATHER THAN WHY

Man is both so perfectible and corruptible that he can go mad by means of his reason.

G. C. Lichtenberg, *The Little Book of Consolation*

The second heresy of strategic therapy is that the therapist should focus not on the analysis of the deeply rooted or on research into the causes of a problem extrapolated from hidden truths, but rather on the nature of the difficulties facing a patient, couple, or family now, and on how they can be changed. What matters is process rather than content, the knowledge of how rather than why. The role of the therapist is to help the patient resolve the present problem and acquire, through this experience, the capacity to adequately confront problems in the future.

The first step is to break the spell. Then the patient learns how to avoid being trapped again by other spells or perceptions and dysfunctional actions. The foundation for this lies in studies and theories that relate to the spontaneous appearance or deliberate realization of change (Watzlawick et al. 1967, 1974). So it is important to give particular attention to one's perception of reality and to the pragmatic aspects of one's relationship with such reality; to how, by means of these processes, problem situations arise; and finally, to how it is possible, through these same processes, to resolve such problem situations.

Our fundamental assumption is that mental and behavioral disturbances are determined by the patient's perception of reality; by the way the patient perceives (or, better, constructs) a reality, then reacts to it with dysfunctional behavior, or so-called psychopathology. The patient usually believes such behavior to be the best way of dealing with a specific situation. That is to say, frequently it is the "attempted solution" that prolongs or aggravates the problem (Nardone 1996, Watzlawick et al. 1974).

The therapeutic intervention is represented by the shift from the patient's point of view, from its original rigid and dysfunctional perceptive-reactive position, to an elastic perspective, with more perceptive-reactive possibilities. We return here to the ethical imperative established by Foerster: "Act always so as to increase the number of choices" (1984, p. 60). This change in perspective produces a change in the perception of reality, which in turn changes reality itself—the entire situation and the patient's reactions to it.

The patient's perceptions become flexible, and thus can be utilized to confront problematic situations without rigidity and persistent error. The patient acquires the capacity to generate a diversity of possible resolutions or strategies when faced with a problem and to begin working toward a solution with the application of the one that appears most likely to effect change. The patient is able to continue the process until a solution is achieved. As Nietzsche stated, "Everything that is absolute pertains to pathology"; thus a solution that is successful in one specific situation, when applied to another, can become a complication in the second problem. In fact, the rigid perceptive-reactive system of a troubled person often expresses itself in the obstinate effort to utilize a strategy that seems to resolve the problem, or that in the past did resolve a similar difficulty but now actually reinforces it.

A rigid perceptive-reactive system can lead to the use of one or more "good solutions" being indiscriminately applied to different problems, with the obvious result that the problems are not only not solved but are complicated by the patient's growing lack of confidence that they can ever be modified. It may seem strange and paradoxical, but often a person's efforts to change either maintain the situation unchanged or increase its complexity. In either case, the person behaves like the drunk who was looking under a lamppost for a key that he had lost. A helpful passerby offered to help him find it. After searching unsuccessfully for quite a while under the lamppost, the helpful gentleman turned to the drunk, a bit annoyed, and asked, "But are you sure that you lost it here?" The other fellow replied, "No, but where I lost it, it is too dark."

The first therapeutic action that must be undertaken is to soften the patient's rigid reactive system by breaking down both the attempted solutions, which sustain the problem, and the tangle of interpersonal reactions related to them to obtain strategies that can be both problem oriented (Fisch et al. 1982, Garcia and Witzaele 1993, Nardone and Watzlawick 1993, Watzlawick et al. 1974,

Weakland 1993, Weakland and Ray 1995, Weakland et al. 1974) and solution oriented (Berg, 1985, Berg and de Shazer 1993, de Shazer 1975, 1982a,b, 1985, 1988a,b, 1991, 1993, 1994). Then the therapist and client can work toward a cognitive redefinition of both the situation and its effect on the subject.

THIRD HERESY:
THE THERAPIST IS RESPONSIBLE

To put reality to the test, one must make it walk a tightrope, and one can judge it only insofar as it becomes acrobatic.

Oscar Wilde, *The Artist as Critic*

A theory about the persistence and the change of human problems that is radically different from classical psychological and psychiatric conceptions leads to procedures (strategies designed to provoke change) and processes (the evolving phases of change) that are also completely different from classical forms of psychotherapy. At the therapeutic levels of both procedure and process, the strategic approach is the result of the application to the clinical field of the theory of logical types, developed by Whitehead and Russell (1910–1913) in their *Principia Mathematica* of the modern mathematical logic concerning "self-deception logic," "the logic of belief" and the logic of "self-fulfilling prophecies" (Da Costa 1989a,b, Grana 1990), as well as the evolution of strategic logic models (Elster 1985), indicating the methods to set up both rigorous and elastic problem-solving processes. It also draws on systems theory and cybernetics (Ashby 1954, 1956, Bateson 1967, 1972, Bateson et al. 1956, 1964, Foerster 1974b, Wiener 1967). It is based on the conception of circular causality, the recursion between cause and effect, and the principle of the discontinuity of change and growth.

From this perspective, the usual conviction that problems that mature over a long period of time necessitate an equally lengthy period of treatment, or that great suffering and complicated situations require a similarly complicated and painful resolution, becomes not only refutable but devoid of meaning. To resolve a pathology effectively, we need to change its actual persistency, and not its past formation, by means of an intervention capable of breaking down its balance and reorienting the patient toward a new perception of reality. Such a type of intervention does not require a lot of time and great suffering but only well-planned and well-applied therapeutic strategies, as more than thirty years of brief therapy applications have shown (Asay and Lambert 1999, Bloom 1995).

However, it is important to state that we are convinced that a pathological system cannot find the solution to a problem within itself, without running into recursiveness, that is, producing only a so-called first-order, rather than a second-order, change. These are two types of change: one that occurs within a given system, which itself remains unchanged, and one whose occurrence changes the system itself. To exemplify this distinction in more behavioral terms, a person having a nightmare can do many things in his dream, such as run, hide, fight, scream, jump off a cliff, but no change from any one of these behaviors within the world of the dream would ever terminate the nightmare. We shall refer to this kind of change as first-order change. The one way out of the nightmare involves a change from dreaming to waking. Waking is no longer a part of the dream, but a change to an altogether different state. This kind of change is a second-order change (Watzlawick et al. 1974). The basis of our strategic approach and a full discussion of its theoretical foundation are presented in Watzlawick and colleagues (1974).

There may be no better example of the strategic approach to the solution of problems (and of its fundamental difference from other forms of psychotherapy) than the famous "nine-dot problem." The problem is to link the nine dots in Figure 3–1 by four straight lines without lifting the pencil from the page. The reader who has never encountered this puzzle should draw the pattern of dots on a piece of paper and try to solve the problem before reading on and, most important, before looking at the solution.

Almost everybody who first tries to solve this problem introduces as part of his problem solving an assumption that makes the solution impossible. The assumption is that the dots compose a square and that the solution must be found within that square—a self-imposed condition that the instructions do not contain. One's failure, therefore, does not lie in the impossibility of the task, but in the attempted solution. Having now created the problem, it does not matter in the least which combination of four lines he now tries, and in what order; he always finishes with at least one unconnected dot. This means that he can run through the totality of the first-order change possibilities existing within the square but will not solve the task. The solution is a second-order change, which consists in leaving the field and which cannot be contained within itself because, in the language

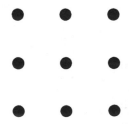

Figure 3–1. The nine-dot problem.

of *Principia Mathematica*, it involves all of a collection and cannot, therefore, be part of it (Watzlawick et al. 1974).

To resolve the problem of the nine points, the subject must step outside the logical schema that traps him inside the square. Very few people manage to solve the nine-dot problem by themselves. Those who fail and give up are usually surprised at the unexpected simplicity of the solution (Figure 3–2). The analogy between this and many a real-life situation is obvious. We have all found ourselves in comparable boxes, and it did not matter whether we tried to find the solution calmly and logically or, as is more likely, ended up running frantically around in circles. But, as mentioned already, it is only from inside the box, in the first-order change perspective, that the solution appears as a surprising flash of enlightenment beyond our control. In the second-order change perspective it is a simple change from one set of premises to another of the same logical type. The one set includes the rule that the task must be solved within the [assumed] square; the other does not. In other words, the solution is found as a result of examining the assumptions about the dots, not the dots themselves. Or, to make the same statement

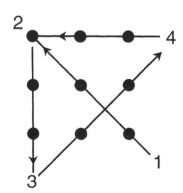

Figure 3–2. Solution to the nine-dot problem.

in more philosophical terms, it obviously makes a difference whether we consider ourselves as pawns in a game whose rules we call reality or as players of the game who know that the rules are "real" only to the extent that we have created or accepted them, and we can change them (Watzlawick et al. 1974).

It may be useful to compare this kind of problem solving and change with the assumptions that are at the root of most classical schools of psychotherapy. It is generally held that change comes about through insight into the past causes of the present trouble. But, as the nine-dot problem exemplifies, there is no cogent reason for this excursion into the past; the genesis of the self-defeating assumption that precedes the solution is quite irrelevant; the problem is solved in the here and now by stepping outside the "box." There is increasing awareness among clinicians that while insight may provide very sophisticated explanations of a symptom, it does little if anything to change it for the better. This empirical fact raises an important epistemological issue. All theories have limitations that follow logically from their premises. In the case of psychiatric theories, these limitations are more often than not attributed to human nature. For instance, within the psychoanalytic framework, symptom removal without the solution of the underlying conflict responsible for the symptom must lead to symptom substitution. This is not because this complication lies in the nature of the human mind; it lies in the nature of the theory, that is, in the conclusions that follow from its premises (Watzlawick et al. 1974).

From this perspective, human problems can be resolved by means of specific strategies that break the feedback loops that maintain the problem. Change in the patient's behavior and insight follow from this breakdown of a dysfunctional equilibrium, because change depends on modification of the perceptive-reactive system— or the view of reality—that is actively maintained by the attempted solutions applied by the patient. The patient must be "forced" to abandon his rigid perspective and be led to other possible perspectives that can bring about new realities and new solutions, as in the example of the nine-dot problem.

To achieve such a result, one need not search for a presupposed original trauma, the removal of which would solve the patient's problems; neither is a slow and progressive acquisition of insight indispensable to the search for self-consciousness. These are procedures based on assumptions of a linear causality of a deterministic relationship between cause and effect, as well as conceptions and convictions, among others, which have been overcome by modern science, from biology to physics.

Instead of linear assumptions, what is needed are direct and indirect behavior prescriptions, nonordinary logic interventions, suggestions, and reframing. They break through the rigidity of the relational and cognitive system that maintains the problem situation and they complete the indispensable logical leap that opens up new ways of change, making possible both personal growth and a new psychological equilibrium. As Milton Erickson affirms (Watzlawick et al. 1974):

> Psychotherapy is sought not primarily for enlightenment about the unchangeable past but because of dissatisfaction with the present and a desire to better the future. In what direction and how much change is needed neither the patient nor the therapist can know. But a change in the current situation is required, and once established, however small, necessitates other minor changes, and a snowballing effect of these minor changes leads to other more significant changes in accord with the patient's potentials. Whether the changes are evanescent, permanent, or evolve into other more significant changes is of vital importance in any understanding of human behavior for the self and others. I have viewed much of what I

have done as expediting the current of change already seething within the person and family—but currents that need the "unexpected," the "illogical," and the "sudden" move to lead them into tangible fruition. [p. ix]

In this absolutely heretical approach the therapist assumes the responsibility of directly influencing the behavior and worldview of the patient. To this end, in the interests of the patient, the therapist uses communicative strategies and other means of effecting change. This point will be dealt with at length in Chapter 4, but for the moment all that is necessary is to clarify these points:

1. In strategic therapy, the therapist maintains the initiative in all that takes place during the course of treatment and applies a specific technique to deal with each particular problem. For the therapist, the first question must always be, Which strategy functions best in a given case?

2. If a specific therapy is functioning correctly, certain indicators of change should appear early on in the treatment. If this is not the case, most likely the intervention chosen is not appropriate and must be superseded with another that is more successful.

3. The therapist must possess a mental elasticity and a wide repertory of strategies and techniques that, as we shall see, stem from orientations different from those of the classical schools of psychotherapy. There must be room to shift gears when the facts make it clear that one is far from the desired goal, and to study ad hoc strategies so that techniques already successfully utilized in similar cases can be creatively modified. As we have been stressing, the therapist needs to adapt the treatment to the patient, not the patient to the treatment.

FOURTH HERESY:
CHANGE COMES BEFORE INSIGHT

It is much more difficult to do a thing than to talk about it.

Oscar Wilde, *The Artist as Critic*

Another heresy at the level of strategies and processes of change lies in the fact that most psychotherapies, imbued with the idea of cogito-centrism (the centrality of thought in respect to action), have as their point of departure the presupposition that action follows from thought. Consequently, to change distorted behavior or a problematical situation, the patient's thinking must change first; hence, the necessity of insight, of procedures to analyze the mind, and all those techniques based on "consciousness raising" and "rationalization" of action.

In strategic therapy based on radical constructivism, this process is inverted. We believe that in order to change a problem situation one must first change the action and then change the patient's thinking—or, better, the point of view or "frame of reality." Foerster and his aesthetic imperative again come to mind in this regard.

It is our concrete experience that determines any change in our manner of perceiving and reacting to reality. We believe that the entire work of Jean Piaget clearly demonstrates how the acquisition of new knowledge occurs through a process that moves from *experience to cognition*. Only after change—or the new experience—is achieved does cognition allow it to be repeated and reapplied at will.

We do not, therefore, want to negate the influence of thought and cognition on action, but we do wish to emphasize that change of a perceptive-reactive situation must originate first in concrete experience; only after that can it become cognitive knowledge. By *experience* we do not mean the reductive physical concept of sensori-motor action, but rather that which we all perceive in our relations with others and with the world. A strong emotion determined by a relation or communication with another person may be an example of a new, concrete situation and can shift the patient's outlook on reality. A casual disruption in our usual routine or a strong suggestion are other examples of concrete experiences that can change our frame of reality.

The strategic therapist, therefore, is oriented pragmatically to action and to the rupture of dysfunctional feedbacks that the patient experiences within, with others, and with the world. The aim is to effect this change by bringing about concrete perceptive-reactive experiences. The therapist first seeks to produce modifications of the patient's perceptive-reactive faculty and then to pass on to redefinitions, at the cognitive level, of that which is experienced, in a pragmatic synthesis of the therapist's influence and the patient's continuous wish for autonomy. From this perspective, any attempt to produce insight at the early stage of therapy is considered to be a counterproductive maneuver insofar as it increases resistance to change. Every system, according to the principle of homeostasis, resists any alteration of itself. As we shall see, the rupture of the perceptive-reactive system and attempted solutions must usually occur without the patient's awareness of the process, so as to obviate resistance. Only after successfully effecting the change can the therapist explain the "tricks" or the "benevolent lies" utilized.

To make clearer the differences between the ways procedure and process are used in strategic therapy and in other approaches, let us use a clinical example: Confronted with an agoraphobic patient, traditional psychotherapy would begin by exploring the origin of the patient's fear and its causes in the past. Then the patient would be led, by means of rationalization and explanation, to confront the fear and its triggers. Normally, this procedure requires many months or even years.

In strategic therapy, a patient may be asked to perform some embarrassing task when experiencing attacks of anxiety or panic, with the usual result that the person comes to the next appointment feeling guilty for not having carried out the assignment but, oddly, also noting that in the interim the symptoms that brought the person to therapy have not recurred. By means of a "benevolent lie" that leads the person to behave differently, the rigid system of perception that had restricted the patient to a symptomatic response is shattered. From that point on, the person, whether aware of it or not, has experienced mastery of what had seemed an overwhelming fear, and the treatment begins to make progress. Through a concrete personal experience, the patient has acquired faith in the possibility of modifying the situation.

To return to the initial concept, it is action or experience that produces change, which is then strengthened and made conscious. Strategic therapy, then, can be seen as a chess game played between therapist and patient. After each "change" or result, one proceeds to a redefinition of change itself. The therapeutic program develops strategy after strategy, based on the effects observed in the effort, to apply the most efficacious treatment for a specific problem or a specific phase of therapy.

In a chess game, particular combinations of moves and countermoves follow from a specific opening made by one player. In therapy, there are particular strategic programs for specific types of problems (in Chapter 5 we shall give several examples). Often the therapist must creatively modify the system of foreseeable moves by finding new, unexpected, and apparently illogical strategies that take into account the whole gamut of possible combinations, thus amplifying the complexity of the game and its possibilities. Thus the strategic approach is not a simple series of effective "recipes," but a prospect for confronting human problems. It is not concerned with extinguishing all problems in the life of the patient, but with finding solutions to the specific problem that the patient is coping with at this time. The idea is not to apply magical tricks, but rather to creatively adapt to each particular individual and context logical principles concerning the formation and solution of problems.

The process of therapy closes with the "checkmate" of the problem presented at its outset, and with the patient's acquisition of the "procedures" to autonomously play and win this specific sort of game. "For the rest," says Bateson (1972), "to live is to play a game whose purpose is to discover the rules, which are always changing and always undiscoverable" (pp. 19–20).

4

CLINICAL PRACTICE

I certainly can't say that change is always for the better;
but what I can say is that improvement necessitates change.

G. C. Lichtenberg, *The Little Book of Consolation*

Before we examine the clinical application of our approach to therapy, it will be useful to review a few of its basic concepts. The relationship between therapists and patients in strategic therapy is not a sort of paid friendship and is far from being a form of consolation or confession. Rather, as we have seen, it is a kind of chess game between therapists on the one hand and patients with their problems on the other. As in chess, there is a set of rules, step-by-step development, and a series of consolidated strategies, each appropriate to a specific situation—all designed to bring a game to a satisfactory conclusion.

This chapter explains the therapeutic process step by step (much as a chess manual explains possible moves), from the first encounter between therapist and patient to the end of treatment. The chapter includes a series of detailed descriptions of both consolidated strategies and therapeutic techniques—analogous to the common opening moves in a chess game. Clearly, we cannot be exhaustive as regards the repertoire of possible strategies, any more than a chess manual can detail all possible moves. The combinations in both cases are infinite, depending on the interaction between the two players.

PROCESSES AND PROCEDURES OF THERAPY

Brief strategic therapy is usually accomplished in ten sessions or less, and is directed at the elimination of symptoms and the resolution of problems. This approach, as will become clear, is not behaviorist in nature, nor is it a superficial, symptom-oriented therapy. As we have said, the success of strategic therapy in resolving a problem lies in breaking the circular reaction system that maintains the problem, redefining the situation, and subsequently changing the patient's perception of the reality that is forcing the adoption of dysfunctional solutions. In this sense, the past and clinical history of the patient serve only to inform the selection of strategies with which to tackle the problem; they do not form the basis per se of the therapeutic procedure, as in the case of psychoanalysis. From the first meeting with the patient, instead of concentrating on the past, the therapist focuses on, and evaluates, the following:

1. What is happening within the three types of the patient's interdependent relationships, namely, with self, with others, and with the world.

2. How the problem presented is perpetuated within those relationship patterns.
3. How the patient has tried so far to solve the problem (what the attempted solution is).
4. How the problem situation can be changed as quickly as possible.

After having formulated one or more hypotheses relating to these four points, and having reached an agreement with the patient(s) regarding the goal of therapy, the therapist can put the various strategies into operation.

If the treatment is effective, there is usually a lessening of the symptoms right from the first session, followed by a progressive change in the patient's way of perceiving self, others, and the world. The patient's rigid perceptual framework, which maintained the problem, gradually becomes more elastic. At the same time, the patient's sense of autonomy and self-esteem increase, along with the realization that solving the problem is now a tangible possibility. The following list of the stages of treatment helps to delineate the processes involved in this form of strategic therapy (adapted from Weakland et al. 1974, and Nardone 1993, 1996):

- First appointment and building of therapeutic relationship
- Definition of the problem
- Agreement on the goals of treatment
- Pinpointing the perceptive-reactive system keeping the problem alive
- Devising therapy and change strategies, and applying and adapting tactics and techniques
- Conclusion of treatment.

Each of these stages will be explored in detail, and specific examples can be found in the case histories in the concluding chapters.

FIRST APPOINTMENT AND BUILDING OF THE THERAPEUTIC RELATIONSHIP

The initial meeting between therapist and patient is of great importance to the therapy as a whole. Aristotle said that a good start was half the job already done. In this opening phase of therapy, the primary goal is to create a positive atmosphere of trust within which the therapist can collect information that will be of use in formulating a diagnosis and preparing the ground for subsequent interventions. Here it is fundamental to learn to speak the patient's language. The therapist must fit into the representational framework of the person seeking help, adapting personal language and actions to the worldview and communicative style of the patient. For example, if the patient is a rational, logical person, the therapist should speak and act in logical and rational ways, with no flights of fancy. If, however, the therapist is confronted with an imaginative and poetic person, then imaginative and creative language—not rigid, logical rationality—will put the therapist in tune with the patient. Clearly, this initial step is completely contrary to the usual psychoanalytic procedures, in which it is the patient who has to learn the language of psychoanalysis and become conversant with its theories in order to benefit from therapy.

This first stage is critical. By accepting what patients communicate about themselves and their problems and by speaking each patient's language, the therapist can create an atmosphere of trust, understanding, and positive influence that will allow "manipulation" and guidance of the patient's actions. In effect, the therapist assumes therapeutic power and overcomes the patient's resistance to change.

In this first contact with the patient, a good therapist stimulates the patient's motivation and trust, giving positive suggestions and leading the patient, without contradicting the patient's convictions, to carry out actions that may be completely at odds with the patient's prior conceptual framework.

DEFINING THE PROBLEM

Successfully resolving the problem and the dysfunctional interactional system by which it is maintained requires that it be clearly and concretely defined. Right from the first session, the therapist must concentrate on the problem itself. Arriving at a pragmatic definition requires not only taking into consideration the patient's personal observations but also eliciting from the patient the clearest possible explanation of the problem. This process can take some time, as people often are not good at describing their problems clearly, and it may become necessary to look more closely at what the patient is experiencing in order to help define the problem and move on to the practical part of the treatment. That this process can be time-consuming should not worry the therapist unduly, because the sessions spent in clarifying the problem, if conducted in the patient's own communicative style, constitute a form of therapeutic intervention. Even as early as this exploratory stage, it is not unusual to see symptoms improve. The famous Hawthorne effect, well known to social psychologists, describes this phenomenon exactly (Mayo 1933): simply knowing that someone is concerned can positively influence the situation. Moreover, a clear and concrete definition of the problem is of great help in finding the fastest and most effective solution, and thus time spent in the so-called diagnostic phase will be made up for later.

In defining and evaluating the problem, the therapist should bear in mind a few general characteristics of human problems that will help in the definition of specific situations. Greenberg (1980) formulated two categories of human problems: (1) a person's relationship with himself, and (2) a person's relationship with others. We would like to add a third category: (3) a person's relationship with the world, that is, with the social environment—the values and norms of the social context within which the person lives.

In our view, if difficulties arise in one of these relationship areas, the others are also affected. In fact, all three types of relationship, which are components of the existence of every individual, influence each other and interact interdependently.

What seems to be most important in this problem-solving and solution-oriented therapy is to establish how this circularity of interdependence works and whether problems in one of the three relationship dimensions are more keenly felt by the patient than those in the others. In such a case, the dimension in question would provide the ideal starting point for interventions through which the whole dysfunctional perceptive-reactive system could eventually be changed.

To arrive at a concrete definition of the problem, the therapist needs to be able to answer the following questions:

- What are the patient's usual, observable behavior patterns?
- How does the patient define the problem?
- How does the problem manifest itself?
- In whose company does the problem appear, worsen, disguise itself, or not appear?
- Where does it usually appear or not appear?
- In what situations?

- How often does the problem appear and how serious is it?
- What has been done and is currently being done (by the patient alone or by others) to resolve the problem?
- Whom or what does the problem benefit?
- Who could be hurt by the disappearance of the problem?

Having answered these questions, the therapist is able to select and put into effect the appropriate strategies aimed at breaking the vicious circle of action and reaction that maintains the problem.

AGREEMENT ON THE GOALS OF THERAPY

The necessity of defining the goals of therapy may appear obvious, but we consider it of great pragmatic importance for two main reasons: (1) it is a guide for the therapist in that it gives the therapy a specific direction, and allows a progressive evaluation of the results achieved; (2) for the patient, defining the goals of therapy is a positive suggestion, and the discussion of and agreement on the duration and the aims of the treatment can reinforce and enhance the patient's willingness to cooperate and commit to a successful outcome. The patient therefore feels actively involved and in control of the therapeutic process. Moreover, in agreeing on the goals to be reached, the therapist is, in fact, signaling a message to the patient: "I believe you are fully capable of reaching this goal" or "I believe that you will manage to solve your problems." This type of message greatly encourages change and generally motivates the patient to cooperate.

Rosenthal (1966), in his famous experiments, demonstrated the influence of experimenters on the experiments they conduct. Experimenters influence, through their expectations, the behavior and efficiency of the experimental objects, be they mice or human beings. Positive expectation on the part of the experimenter can greatly improve a subject's performance. The same holds for hypnotherapy: if the hypnotherapist expresses certainty that the subject will go into a trance, the subject, in fact, will most likely do so.

Finally, in agreeing on the goals of therapy and in planning to achieve them, it is most important that the therapist not exert too much pressure and thereby provoke anxiety in the patient, but rather engage the patient in a gradual progression of preliminary smaller goals. The patient must not feel forced to change, but instead should see the treatment as systematic and thorough, with concrete aims. If the patient feels rushed, the risk is great that the treatment will go awry. It has in fact been shown that, paradoxically, encouraging patients to take their time and go slowly often brings about a change more readily, while attempting to hurry the process along slows down change by reinforcing the patient's resistance. The patient may even become too intimidated to continue the treatment.

IDENTIFYING THE PERCEPTIVE-REACTIVE SYSTEM MAINTAINING THE PROBLEM

With the first three phases of treatment completed, the therapist must study the patient's situation carefully to determine the key aspects that sustain the problem. Looked at another way, the therapist must determine the best strategy to bring about change. Thus, over and above clarifying the problem, the therapist must also understand how it is maintained and on which of the factors to act to ensure success.

Clinical experience has shown that, ironically, it is often the patient's very attempts to solve the problem that maintain it. The attempted solution becomes the true problem. As in the old joke recounted earlier, about the drunk searching for his key, the thing that makes the whole situation problematical is not his having lost the key in the first place, which is not a pathological act, but rather the drunk's attempted solution of looking for the key under the street lamp, knowing full well that he had not lost the key there. His insistence on searching in the wrong place is the problem. Often patients' attempted solutions become "generalized" and transferred to other situations, which then, too, become problematical. In these cases, in order to bring about change, the therapist must intervene at the level of these attempted solutions, singling out the most fundamental self-reinforcing pattern for direct therapeutic intervention.

At this stage of therapy, the therapist should also carefully evaluate the influence a patient's social interactions may have on attempted solutions. The therapist may deem it necessary to intervene directly in these interpersonal relationships, as well as in the attempted solutions, or maybe to concentrate solely on the reorganization of that relationship system, given that the attempted solutions will be influenced in turn by the change in the relationship system as a whole.

The therapist must judge each case individually, deciding whether it would be more effective to intervene at the level of the dysfunctional perceptive-reactive system of the individual, inducing a chain reaction that can affect interpersonal relationships, or whether it would be preferable to extend the therapy to include more subjects and tackle the problem at the level of the patient's family relationships, where changes may in turn alter the perceptive-reactive system of the identified patient.

As pointed out earlier, the therapist needs to decide which type of relationship (the patient's relationship with self, with others, or with the world) provides the best starting point for therapeutic intervention. The appropriate treatment, indirectly or directly systemic, should be chosen. To repeat a key point: instead of investigating presumed intrapsychic factors or presumed past trauma, the therapist is interested in the patient's concrete actions in the here and now and in the interpersonal and social reactions to these actions. Clearly, a person's actions are influenced mainly by emotions and conceptions of reality, but we believe, as we have already stated, that these, too, only change as a result of concrete experience. Thus, when determining what it is that maintains the problem, and when applying the strategies for change, it must be remembered that therapy must induce a concrete experience of change. If therapists have correctly followed the phases of treatment to this stage, they should now be in a position both to identify the most effective interventions and to improvise and apply the appropriate strategies.

THERAPY PROGRAMMING AND STRATEGIES OF CHANGE

Before we consider specific therapeutic procedures, we need to state our belief that it is not legitimate to examine therapeutic strategies out of the context—the particular case—in which they have been developed and used. This is because patient–therapist communication and interaction also contribute to change. The simple fact that patient and therapist communicate at all can sometimes produce therapeutic effects.

In that the process of therapy itself is a therapeutic strategy, our distinction between processes and procedures is a purely linguistic one; in reality these two components of the therapeutic process are indivisible.

The most effective strategies are based on the fundamental axiom of the strategic approach, namely, that it is the therapy that must adapt itself to the patient, not the patient to the therapy. With this in mind, in preparing an approach, the therapist will use strategies that have previously been effective in similar cases, but will choose or improvise procedures for every individual case. For example, the same general strategy may have to be applied in radically different ways, depending on specific social and cultural factors and the personality traits of the patient.

As we have said previously, the therapist must learn the patient's language and representational system in order to present interventions in a way that the patient can readily accept. Thus, a particular form of therapy will never be precisely the same for all patients, but will be modified according to the particular perceptive and communication styles of each individual. In addition, if a strategy proves ineffective, it must be rapidly replaced or supplemented by others.

At this early stage of treatment it is also quite useful to bear in mind that change is much more likely to come about as a result of insisting on apparently minor or even trivial issues and on seemingly unimportant details. In this way patients will not have the impression that excessive demands are made on their capacities and resources, and this, too, is likely to decrease resistance to change. In effect, such seemingly minor and indirect interventions may have far greater effects than imagined.

Such small changes in a system's functioning may set off a chain reaction that will, in the end, restore the system's balance. Thus, even seemingly banal or insignificant changes may have great power and should be made full use of in therapy. When, through a gradual progression of small-scale changes, the therapist has brought a person to the point of modifying dysfunctional actions and images of the world, the therapy has achieved its goal.

Finally, before going on to describe the therapeutic procedures in detail, it is essential to realize that their effectiveness depends not purely and simply on their specific validity for particular symptoms or problems, but above all on the personal influence and charisma of the therapist—a factor that we hold to be a principal determinant of success and failure. The effectiveness of a strategy depends heavily on the suggestive framework within which it is presented to the patient. Presented correctly, it can lead to full (and often involuntary) therapeutic cooperation and thus to a willingness to change (Frank 1973).

To create this framework of suggestions, the therapist has to learn to utilize what we referred to at the beginning of this book as "injunctive language" (after Brown) and "performative speech acts" (after Austin). This type of therapeutic communication, of which Erickson's hypnotic techniques have been the best examples to date, is fundamental to strategic therapy. It is what we call hypnotherapy without trance. In using it, the therapist adopts procedures similar to hypnotic suggestions to bring about change. The recurrent therapeutic procedures utilized in this approach can be divided into two types: actions and therapeutic communication, and behavioral prescriptions.

ACTIONS AND THERAPEUTIC COMMUNICATION

Learning to Speak the Patient's Language

The first thing the therapist attempts to do is to learn to use the patient's language. This key communication technique derives from Ericksonian hypnotherapy (Erickson 1952, 1954a,b, 1958, 1964, 1965, 1980, Erickson and Rossi 1975, 1977, 1979, 1983, Erickson et al. 1979), at least as far as its application in psychotherapy is concerned. Erickson employed communication methods that he had used in trance induction as therapeutic language. In fact, in trance induction, he imitated the patient's perceptive and communicative style, slowly and gradually taking control, until finally persuading the patient to let go and fall into a trance.

Bandler and Grinder (1975b) defined this communication strategy as the "tracing technique." They had studied Erickson's communication techniques and found that in his first encounters with patients he adopted their own style of language and their own personal concepts of reality. Furthermore, he even imitated the patients' forms of nonverbal communication in order to put them completely at their ease, which enabled him to gradually influence them with his suggestions and prescriptions.

But it was not Erickson who first discovered the effectiveness of this persuasion technique; it had been an essential component of classical rhetoric for more than two thousand years. Aristotle, for example, in his *Retorica ad Alexandrum*, said, as did the Sophists, that if you want to persuade someone you must use his own arguments. Moreover, experimental psychology has repeatedly shown that human beings are attracted to, and influenced by, things that are familiar to them or similar to themselves. This knowledge is utilized in tangible and often far from noble ways by professionals of mass persuasion.

For many years the social psychologist Robert Cialdini has been studying strategies of persuasion, and in one of his studies of the selling techniques employed by insurance agents he found that clients tend to sign the contract more readily if the agent resembles them in some way: age, religion, ideas, language, and the like (Cialdini 1984). Clients do not realize that salespeople are trained to mimic their language and agree with their views in order to find those points of interpersonal contact that are useful in getting the client to sign on the dotted line. Cialdini also found positive results in his research into the use of these persuasion techniques in winning a person's approval. The success of many advertising campaigns is due to the fact that they reflect the lifestyle and day-to-day language of the target population.

The wealth of such data shows clearly how important it is to adopt communicative techniques that allow the therapist to influence the patient as rapidly as possible. Despite the fact that patients ask for help in changing their problems, they usually, albeit unknowingly, resist change. This resistance can be lessened by using this style of communication. To be effective, however, it must be carried out in as natural a way as possible and must in no way appear artificial; otherwise, it can have the opposite effect. If the patient feels mocked or ridiculed, resistance will increase.

Careful training in communication is essential for success. This training is not dissimilar to that of actors in that therapists have to learn to adapt their own communicative style and repertory of expressions to the broad spectrum of possible clinical situations. This adaptation, or shall we say "performance," must be as natural as possible if it is to be convincing. Therapists in training should have the opportunity to participate in a wide variety of simulated sessions, to have sessions video recorded, and thus to monitor their own progress.

We believe that preparation in communicative facility is excellent for promoting mental agility. By learning to adapt their language to various situations, contexts, and personal styles, therapists also learn to continually shift their perspectives on reality, which is essential if they are to be able to solve the great diversity of human problems they will be presented with.

Reframing

Reframing is one of the more subtle techniques of persuasion. It changes not a person's perception of reality, but rather the meaning it has for him. Putting the same fact into a different context of meaning, and so looking at it from a different perspective, changes its value radically. As we have said many times, reality is determined by a person's worldview; if that perspective changes, "reality" changes, too.

Let us take a historical example. During the fifteenth century the heads of the Catholic Church were confronted by the problem of a pagan water cult that was being practiced in Italy. The local people believed that several of their freshwater springs had supernatural powers. (See Dini [1980] for explication of the ancient traditions underlying such cults.) The ecclesiastical authorities intervened, trying to stamp out the cult by harshly reprimanding its followers and destroying their shrines. In 1425 Saint Bernard of Siena had soldiers destroy a pagan temple after all his preachings against the cult had been in vain. But even this did not succeed.

At this point, the saint and other churchmen found the solution to the problem, perhaps by remembering what Saint Gregory the Great had done a century before them. They built churches on the sites of the ruined pagan temples and consecrated them to the Virgin Mary, saying that the waters were indeed sacred owing to her presence. In effect, they had reframed popular beliefs in such a way that the cult was no longer at odds with the Church, and the people were therefore free to continue in their conviction that the springs were sacred.

Let us analyze this strategy. In a situation where preaching and violent intervention had been to no avail, a strategic move achieved the desired effect—a move that was in keeping with the popular beliefs but that added one important variable that changed the perceptual perspective of the cult and succeeded in changing it from pagan to Christian. A clinical example of such a move would be the reframing of a phobic person's perception of help. (This approach is described in detail in Chapter 5.) Patients are told that they definitely need, and, in fact, cannot do without, the help of other people. But the therapist intimates, by means of double messages, that such help could aggravate their symptoms. In practice, the therapist redirects the fear that has led the patients to ask for help, and thereby stops the help-seeking behavior.

Reframing can be achieved either purely verbally or by certain actions that lead persons to change their view of reality, just as reframing effects can be produced by means of behavioral prescriptions, which will be examined later. Reframing can vary in complexity, going from a simple cognitive redefinition of an idea or behavior pattern to the use of metaphors and evocative suggestions, and even to complicated paradoxical reframings.

In a general sense, all the therapeutic strategies cited here can be considered reframings in that all are ultimately geared toward changing the patient's behavior and point of view. There are those who maintain that verbal reframing by means of dialogue is the key method employed by all forms of psychotherapy (Simon et al. 1985), changing the "mental map" of a patient being the factor common to all forms of psychotherapy. As far as we are concerned, reframing has nothing to do with the job of attributing meaning to emotions. This persuasive strategy works on the perceptive structure on which the subjective interpretations and behavior are based, rather than directly or mainly on the semantic aspects of reality.

At the semantic level, the strategic therapist offers neither reassurance nor confirmation of the meaning of things, but, on the contrary, raises doubts that break the patient's habitual perceptive-reactive rigidity, creating chinks in the patient's cognitive and behavioral armor. Newton Da Costa, a logician at the University of São Paulo, in Brazil, has shown how the raising of doubt regarding the logical rational explanation is particularly effective in unhinging rigid mental structures. Da Costa maintains that in convincing persons to change their opinions, it is much more effective to plant doubts about the logic of their reasoning than to demonstrate fully and rationally the incorrectness or inadequacy of their ideas or behavior (personal communication, 1989).

Doubt can be likened to a woodworm that gets inside a piece of wood and devours it from the inside. Doubt grows by devouring the preexisting logic that surrounds it. Doubt mobilizes the system's entropy, starting a slow but devastating chain reaction, which can lead to changes in the whole system. Therefore, we believe, along with Simon and colleagues (1985), that reframing a person's "mental map" is the goal of all psychotherapy, but reframing in the strategic approach is completely different from the pursuit of insight that is typical of other therapeutic approaches.

Moreover, the art of reframing as a technique of persuasion is certainly not a new discovery and does not even have its origins in the therapeutic field; it, too, was a commonly used intervention in classical rhetoric, above all by the Sophists, renowned masters of the verbal art of persuasion. Returning to more recent times, however, social psychology research has shown that a person's perceptions and reactions can be changed, not by directly altering the rational meaning attributed to things, but instead by using reframing techniques.

Perhaps the best experimental demonstration of the enormous power that certain suggestions have to induce change is supplied by E. J. Langer, a psychologist at the University of California. Standing in a line of people waiting to use a photocopier in the library, a female student asked if she might go ahead of the others, and, depending on the exact wording of her request, got very different reactions from the other students. When she said, "Excuse me. I've got five pages. May I use the photocopier because I'm in a real hurry?" 95 percent of the students let her go ahead. By contrast, only 60 percent consented when she said, "Excuse me, I've got five pages. May I use the photocopier?" At first glance, it seems that the added explanation "because I'm in a hurry" was all-important. But a third version of the request showed that this was not exactly the case. Here, "because" was included, but nothing else was added: "Excuse me, I've got five pages. Can I use the photocopier because I've got to make the copies?" In this case, 83 percent of the people asked agreed, even though they were given no additional information about the request that might have prompted their acquiescence. Just as the "chip, chip" of the turkey chick triggers an automatic reaction from its mother, even when the chick is simply a stuffed imitation, so the word *because* triggered automatic agreement in Langer's subjects, even when no reason was actually given (Cialdini 1984).

This experiment shows how a person's reactions to a situation can be modified if the situation is reframed, not necessarily in a logical or rational way. It also shows the power of certain suggestive forms of communication to lessen resistance and confuse logical-rational convictions. Thus reframing is not a direct means of attributing meaning, but a way of softening a person's rigid logic. It opens new horizons and possibilities for changing the seeming immutability of a person's mindset.

When the therapist restructures a patient's reality, imitating the latter's ways of interpreting the environment, the therapist must lead the patient to see things from different points of view. Suggestion, elements of classical rhetoric, and logical paradoxes can be utilized, all of which, if used correctly, can alter a person's meaning of the perception of reality, if only for a moment.

Avoiding Negative Formulations

The third strategy of therapeutic communication is directly connected to the first two; in fact, one could say that it punctuates them. Clinical practice has shown that negative formulations regarding a person's behavior or ideas are perceived as blame and only provoke resistance. In hypnosis, negative formulations have a similar effect, and therefore the hypnotherapist tends to rephrase all negative ideas into positive statements. Instead of criticizing a patient's behavior, even when it is clearly dysfunctional, it is far more productive to go along with the patient, making him or her feel at ease, and then to offer suggestions as to how to change the behavior.

For example, faced with two overprotective parents who, by their excessive concerns, have made their son insecure and psychologically fragile, the therapist might compliment them on having dealt so well with a difficult child, and on all the sacrifices they have made in order to protect him from possible dangers in the outside world. The therapist might say, "And, seeing that you have done such a good job so far, I'm sure you will manage admirably to do even better now, in getting him to assume his responsibilities." At this point the therapist would prescribe radically different actions and behavior for the parents. In this way, instead of blaming the parents for the mistakes they have made in bringing up their child and for their suffocating overprotection, and instead of saying to them "Don't do this, don't do that, you've done this wrong and that wrong," the therapist makes use of the parents' capacity to intervene, reframing it positively and giving a direct prescription as to the correct and functional parental behavior that will resolve the problem.

This example combines three different techniques: avoidance of negative formulations, reframing, and prescription. Such techniques generally promote participation and cooperation, even in rigidly difficult patients, and circumvent any negative reactions that blaming the patient might cause. Patients show that they know their actions are dysfunctional by asking for help; there is no need for the therapist to emphasize this.

USE OF PARADOX AND OF PARADOXICAL COMMUNICATION PATTERNS

A logical paradox is a statement that is both true and false, correct and incorrect. The classical example is that of the Cretan Epimenides, who said, "All Cretans are liars." Thus the logic trap is constructed, whether true or false, correct or incorrect. In interpersonal communication, such a paradox occurs when there are two logically inconsistent messages within the same communication. The receiver of the message is in the same predicament as anyone wishing to decide whether Epimenides is telling the truth.

We maintain that the use of paradox is a keystone in therapy, and often extraordinarily effective in rigid perceptive-reactive situations and circular patterns of self-reinforcing behavior. For this reason, this therapeutic procedure plays a fundamental role in the strategic approach. Paradox unhinges the Aristotelian logic of true and false and the Manichean world of opposites (black/ white, beautiful/ugly, correct/incorrect) used as categories to describe reality. As far as the philosophy of knowledge is concerned, logical paradox has undermined every attempt to imprison reality within a descriptive and interpretive system of absolute logic.

Applied to the specific therapeutic context, paradox can break the vicious circle of repetitive behavior that constitutes an attempted solution—the self-reinforcing behavior pattern from which the patient cannot, or is unwilling to, extricate himself. Paradox undermines the patient's preexisting system of perceptions and reactions regarding reality.

Historically speaking, paradox first entered therapy as a therapeutic strategy under the auspices of Viktor Frankl's (1960) "paradoxical intention." But it was really Bateson and colleagues (1956) who first systematically formulated paradox for use in solving problems. They showed that paradox is a basic constituent of mental problems and can be used effectively in their resolution. In other words, they applied the age-old medical dictum *similia similibus curantur* ("like is cured by like").

Paradox appears in various formulations in therapy from paradoxical prescriptions to paradoxical actions and communications. We believe the following examples explain better than any formal analysis can how therapeutic paradoxes work. The first example is of a person who in classical psychiatric terminology would be considered an obsessive hypochondriac, convinced that she is suffering from a serious, incurable disease. Despite conventional medical evidence to the contrary, she persists in this observation and interprets every bodily change that may be a little out of the ordinary as a symptom of her mysterious illness. She is terrified and seeks reassurance and help from everyone around her, and in particular from her therapist. The following is the transcript of a brief conversation with this patient:

> *Patient*: Doctor, I'm exhausted. I feel so ill! I'm so scared! There's something malignant inside me, I can feel it growing. I'm going to die soon! Nobody believes that I'm seriously ill. I sweat all the time, and I can feel my heart beating so fast. And then, you know, as I told my husband, I feel as if there's a curse on me. You won't believe these things, but it's true. Nobody believes me, but it's eating away my insides.

> *Therapist*: Hmmm. (Looking serious and pensive) I really do believe you are seriously ill. In fact, I'm sure that your disease is quite rare. You know there are "curses" and "curses," and it looks as though you've been cursed. (Brief pause.) Yes, I really do feel that you will become very ill, and get worse and worse. In fact, looking at you now, it seems that you're getting worse right here in front of me. You feel ill, right? You look to me as if you are going to feel really bad soon. (Faint smile.)
>
> *Patient*: But doctor, what are you saying, that I'm going to die? So, it's really true, then. I am seriously ill. But, doctor, why haven't all those medical tests I've had done shown anything wrong with me? But are you really sure of what you're saying, that I am ill and that you can really see that someone has put a curse on me?
>
> *Therapist*: But of course. (Slight smile.)
>
> *Patient*: But, doctor, you're making fun of me. I hardly feel ill at all now. In fact, talking to you, I've stopped sweating and I feel much calmer. But, tell me, doctor, how is it that at the age of forty our brains play such tricks on us?

This example shows how, in situations in which rational logic has no effect, paradox can be useful in breaking the repetitive mechanism inherent in obsessions.

Patients are usually worried and surprised when they hear that their terrors are justified. Then, it is they themselves who start to reassure the therapist as to their state of health, saying that the medical tests found nothing wrong. In a few cases, they will smile when they understand the kind trick the therapist has been playing. But the important thing is that the obsessive mechanism of distorted perceptions and reactions has been broken, and their point of view and actions regarding the problem can both begin to change. This example is a good illustration of the logic on which paradoxical intervention is based, and how it is particularly well suited to tackling compulsive acts.

Using this technique, a therapist can create a paradox that renders a symptom voluntary rather than out of the patient's control, but in order to be a symptom, in the strict sense of the word, the problem must be involuntary. From the moment that it becomes voluntary, the symptom completely loses its symptomatic quality. When confronted by such rigid obsessive behavior, rather than analyzing and criticizing, the therapist causes it to escalate to a point where it eliminates itself. The mechanism is the same as that involved in the prescription of the symptom: the destructive capacities of paradox are set in action, and the patient's distorted perceptions are deliberately encouraged. Just as a deliberate attempt to be happy when you are depressed only makes you feel worse, and consciously trying to go to sleep only keeps you awake, leading the patient to persist intentionally in those distorted and seemingly uncontrollable mental processes causes them to lose their essential spontaneity and symptomatic status and they disappear.

Another example of the use of paradox illustrates a slightly different kind of paradoxical action and communication, but reveals the same power of bringing about change. It has to do with those interpersonal situations in which an action and/or an unexpected paradoxical message (a message that could not be foreseen from the usual run of events) turns the situations upside down. The message appears to be neither true nor false and is seemingly at odds with the whole situation, motivating the receiver to make a sudden change in behavior. The enormous effectiveness of such interpersonal communication devices is well illustrated by a strange event that took place in Austria at the end of the 1920s. It received considerable newspaper coverage by virtue of the peculiarities of the case. A young man wishing to commit suicide threw himself off a bridge into the Danube

River. A policeman drawn to the scene by the shouts of the onlook-
ers put his rifle to his shoulder and, aiming it at the young man in the
water, shouted, "Get out, or I'll shoot," at which point the young
man came meekly out of the water, relinquishing his suicide attempt.
In effect, the policeman's action put the youth in a paradoxical situation. The forcible reframing of his reality led him to radical changes
in his behavior and his thought processes. In clinical practice, as in
life in general, such paradoxical experiences, apparently illogical and
completely unforeseen by the patient, rapidly produce that jump in
logic, indispensable for changing a situation.

From these examples it is clear how effective paradoxes can
be in unhinging the rigid, obsessive situations that many patients
create for themselves. The use of paradoxes, albeit in a multitude
of different formats, is particularly effective in the early phase of
strategic therapy, when the therapist has to break the self-reinforcing system of perceptions, actions, and reactions that is maintaining
the patient's problem.

THE UTILIZATION OF RESISTANCE

The utilization of resistance, one of the most refined techniques
derived from the paradox, is of great value in therapy. We believe,
contrary to classical psychoanalytical thinking, that the energy in-
vested in resistance can be redirected so that it can be of great assistance in achieving therapeutic goals. We also recommend that
resistance itself be paradoxically prescribed and thus manipulated.
This is done by creating a therapeutic double bind: the patient's
resistance or rigidity toward the therapist becomes a prescription in
itself, and the patient's subsequent reactions constitute the therapeutic progress. In this way, the primary effect of the resistance is

eliminated, and its underlying energy is put into the service of change; a prescribed resistance, in fact, ceases to be resistance and becomes compliance. Consider this therapist's response to a difficult and distrustful patient. The therapist says, "Look, there is a strong possibility that we can solve your problem, and there are some specific techniques that we could use. But, looking at the circumstances as they stand at the moment, coupled with your outlook on the situation, I don't believe you will succeed." The patient now finds herself in a paradoxical situation. Her usual reaction (her bottled-up aggression toward the therapist) motivates her to do exactly what the therapist said she was incapable of doing. The patient thus collaborates with the therapist, and her resistance is eliminated.

Students of some martial arts learn to use their opponent's strength to their own advantage by combining the natural force of gravity and a sharpened sense of balance. Similarly, this technique redirects the force of the patient's resistance to promote change. The expert hypnotist uses this strategy in reframing a subject's resistance so that she will let herself go into a deeper trance. For example, if the patient resists going into a trance by moving her fingers or her leg, the hypnotist will say, "Very good, your hand [or leg] is responding. Now start to move it faster and faster until you feel tired and really want to rest." Thus, resistance is redefined and its power is directed toward trance induction.

THE USE OF METAPHOR, ANECDOTES, AND STORIES

Other important means of therapeutic communication are the use of metaphor, anecdotes, and stories in recounting events involving other people. These strategies allow the therapist to communicate messages, albeit indirectly, by the identification and projection that people often feel regarding characters and situations in fiction. This technique minimizes resistance because patients are not requested to do anything, nor are their opinions or behavior criticized. The message gets through in disguise, in a manner of speaking. Let us consider an obsessive or phobic patient. To get across to him just how counterproductive it is to listen incessantly to oneself, thereby increasing one's anxiety to the point of a panic attack, a therapist might tell the story of the centipede that, when it started to think how it managed to walk so elegantly with so many legs to move at once, found it could no longer walk at all. The therapist might then get the patient to try the following exercise: "When you leave the room, do what the centipede did: as you walk down the stairs, concentrate on just how difficult it is to keep your balance step after step, putting your foot down in just the right place. Usually, you know, a person starts to stumble and finds he can't walk any farther." This type of tactic is far more effective than giving the patient a scientific explanation. Suggestions are embedded in a story or communicated through metaphors in such a way that the patient is not directly involved, but the evocative power of the story or image counteracts the patient's self-reinforcing conceptions and behaviors.

In strictly linguistic terms, the therapist is making use of the message's "poetic function," that is, the evocative power of these forms of communication (Jakobson 1963). All of us have felt the effects of a particularly touching poem, a passage in a book, or a film. We have felt that we ourselves were really the protagonists; even as we know full well that it is all pretense, our emotions are touched and we live a real and concrete experience. Again, it was Erickson who led the way in inducing this kind of experience in therapy. He brought to psychotherapy what was already known to hypnotists. Indeed, it is usual for a hypnotist to induce a trance by narrating an evocative story that carries suggestions, usually in the form of metaphor. It does not detract from Erickson's originality to note that the power of this persuasion strategy has been used in a variety of contexts for many centuries.

Anyone who is skeptical about the power of evocative language will find it difficult to dismiss what the famous sociologist David Phillips (1974, 1979, 1980) termed the Werther effect. It has a long and interesting history. Goethe's *The Sorrows of Young Werther* recounts the story of a young man who, heartbroken over an ill-fated love affair, commits suicide. Its publication had a shattering effect on the society of the day. Apart from the fame and fortune it earned for Goethe, the book provoked a wave of similar suicides throughout Europe. There were so many in some countries that the authorities banned the book altogether. Phillips's research looks at how the Werther effect manifests itself in modern times—how, for example, a front-page suicide story in a newspaper will dramatically increase the number of suicides among readers of that newspaper. Phillips analyzed suicide statistics in the United States from 1947 to 1968, and found that in the two months following a front-page report of a suicide, there were on average fifty-eight more suicides than normal. Furthermore, there were striking similarities between the subsequent suicides and the original one, in particular with regard to age and social class of the victims.

But Phillips did not stop there. He went on to show that the Werther effect is equally applicable to other events, such as acts of violence and heroism. The only two prerequisites are that the act be publicized and that the receiver either be similar or feel similar to the actor in the original report. Phillips's evidence clearly shows the strength of projection and identification mechanisms, and their power to evoke emulative behavior in receivers of the message who see themselves as similar to the protagonist of a moving story.

Given that psychotherapy is primarily aimed at provoking change in a patient's consciousness and behavior, we must not overlook or underestimate the extraordinary power that can be exercised through the narration of stories and anecdotes that fit in well with the patient's problematical reality. They can lead the patient to make tangible changes in behavior patterns, which in turn can lead to change in perceptive and cognitive makeup.

BEHAVIORAL PRESCRIPTIONS

Behavioral prescriptions are directives that a patient is to follow between sessions. They play a fundamental role in strategic therapy. As we have said, in order to change, one has to undergo concrete experiences; behavioral prescriptions make such concrete experiences of change a reality outside the therapeutic setting.

Behavioral prescriptions merit our particular attention because when patients act alone and in their daily routines they can give themselves the best possible demonstration of their ability to change their problem situations. The fact that they do certain things unknowingly, in response to the therapist's kind tricks, does not change this assertion, because, knowingly or unknowingly, they have still achieved something of which they were previously incapable. Such experiences are the tangible and indisputable proof of the ability to overcome one's difficulties. They clearly open up new perspectives regarding the problem situation; they break the mechanism of actions and reactions and "attempted solutions" that maintain it.

Behavioral prescriptions can be divided into three types: direct, indirect, and paradoxical. *Direct prescriptions* are clear instructions to carry out specific actions. They are aimed at the resolution of the problem or at reaching one of a series of goals on the road to change. This technique is useful for cooperative patients who show little resistance to change. It gives them the key to the resolution of the problem, indicating to them how to act in order to break the mechanism that maintains the problem. Let us consider the case of a man and wife who are continually arguing because, with the best of intentions, each is trying to correct the "bad behavior" of the other. It is easy to see how this simply leads to more and more quarrels. In fact, it becomes a never-ending cycle of actions and reactions.

In such a situation, if just one of the partners becomes more cooperative, it will be sufficient to break the vicious circle of corrections and countercorrections. The therapist need only explain the situation clearly, giving the client the job of breaking the chain, either by not reacting at all to the partner's corrective behavior or by giving the partner the last word.

During the phase immediately following this change in the system that has kept the problem alive, the therapist can use direct prescription to help the patient successfully handle the situations that previously were problematical. To this end, the therapist tells the patient what to do, directly and explicitly, giving a series of step-by-step instructions.

Indirect prescriptions are behavioral injunctions whose real objectives are hidden. The therapist prescribes an action that will produce a different result from the one that was seemingly being specified. This type of prescription utilizes the hypnotic technique of shifting the symptom; usually the patient's attention is drawn to a secondary problem, thereby reducing the intensity of the problem originally presented. As explained in Chapter 3, here we are using nonordinary logic, so that indirect prescription can be devised on the basis of many different typologies of stratagems fitted to break down the specific persistence of the presented problem.

To better explain this technique, let us use the analogy of a magician. The magician draws the audience's attention with some obvious, dramatic movements so that her subtle tricks are not noticed, thus producing a spectacular and seemingly magical effect. Similarly, if the therapist instructs a phobic patient to carry out an anxiety-provoking and embarrassing exercise every time the symptoms manifest themselves, such as writing down in detail the feelings and thoughts that occur at that moment and bringing them to the session, the patient may return ridden with guilt because he has not done what the therapist required. Strangely, he says (and he cannot explain why), he did not suffer any phobic symptoms during the whole week. Obviously, it was either the embarrassment or the anxiety provoked by the exercise that prevented the symptoms from appearing. In other words, his attention was shifted away from the problem itself onto the exercise he was supposed to carry out. This kind trick succeeded in neutralizing the problematical symptoms. But, more important, the patient saw, by means of a concrete experience, that he could control and even eliminate his symptoms. Because they reduce resistance to change by getting the patient to do something without realizing that he is doing it, these interventions play a fundamental role in the first phase of strategic treatment.

Paradoxical prescriptions are a natural progression from the previously described utilization of paradox in therapy. In the case of a seemingly spontaneous and unsolvable problem, such as repetitive obsessions or other particularly resistant dysfunctional behavior, they can be very effective. The patient finds herself in a paradoxical situation, having to perform voluntarily actions that had previously been involuntary and uncontrollable, and that she had always tried to avoid. In this case, also, the voluntary performance of the symptom eliminates it, as it is no longer spontaneous and uncontrollable.

For example, consider the case of a patient who manifested the nightly ritual of checking over and over again that he had turned off all faucets, lights, and gas switches, and that his shoes were exactly placed in a particular position before he could go to sleep. The prescriptions given to this patient were as follows: "Every evening, voluntarily and extremely carefully turn off the lights and the gas switches a specific number of times [see the next chapter for detailed exposition of this technique], using both hands, and position your shoes just as you had always done, but point the shoes in the opposite direction." Within two weeks the nightly rituals ceased. Paradoxical prescriptions, like indirect prescriptions, can be very effective in lessening a patient's resistance to change and are thus of great therapeutic value in the early phases of therapy.

For prescriptions to be followed and to be effective, they need to be very carefully formulated and then presented to the patient almost as hypnotic commands, using the therapeutic communication techniques described above. The use of injunctive or hypnotic language is crucial to their effectiveness in psychotherapy; otherwise, patients rarely carry out the prescriptions they are given, in particular those that are indirect or paradoxical (Watzlawick 1978, Watzlawick and Nardone 1997). This may explain why some therapists complain about the ineffectiveness of prescriptive and paradoxical methods.

Prescriptions must be given to the patient in a slow and repetitive manner at the end of the session. This technique is clearly analogous to hypnotic trance induction. We have seen the effectiveness of behavioral prescriptions in producing change in the therapeutic setting, but what about their effectiveness (in other contexts) as instruments of persuasion? One only has to think of tribal initiation ceremonies that promote social acceptance and that probably go back to the beginnings of humankind. To conclude, however, it is most important that, after a prescription is carried out, the result be examined in detail and the patient praised for progress thus far. The patient should be made aware that problems thought to be insoluble can, in fact, be overcome in a nonstressful way—and that the patient's achievements to date demonstrate this. Prescriptions can be formulated in a variety of ways and may involve very different patterns of behavior; they can be simple tasks to do at home, complicated rituals, or even actions that seemingly have nothing to do with the patient's problem. The important thing is that the therapist use the maximum inventiveness and imagination to find the key to unlock the dysfunctional system of actions and reactions in which the patient is caught.

TERMINATION

The final session in a course of strategic therapy plays an important role. It is the finishing touch, the frame that surrounds the completed painting. The goal is to consolidate the autonomy of the patient. The therapist does this by giving a résumé of the entire course of therapy, explaining in detail the therapeutic process, the strategies used, and the often strange techniques (indirect injunctions, suggestions, paradoxical prescriptions) employed. This final exposé is crucial if the patient is to gain autonomy, to know that the psychic and behavioral reality has changed, thanks to systematic and scientific intervention, and not to some strange form of magic. Above all, it emphasizes how the person tenaciously but unsuccessfully sought the solution of the problem, and that now, having completed this difficult task, the patient is capable of independently dealing with any future problems.

At every stage of the treatment, the therapist tries to avoid creating dependency on the part of the patient. After every small change, the patient must be praised for the hard work and efforts expended in solving the problem. Moreover, right from the beginning, brief therapy induces the patient to assume responsibility for personal actions and, indeed, for the progress of the therapy itself. The therapist's management of the situation and personal influence on the patient are both geared to instill in the patient the capacity to solve the problem as quickly as possible.

Finally, it should be emphasized that, during therapy, it is the qualities and characteristics that already existed within the patient that have been activated and that, after therapy, the patient recognizes and is able to use. Nothing has been added that was not within before. The patient has learned to perceive reality differently and to act accordingly.

5

ADVANCED TECHNIQUES: FROM GENERAL TO SPECIFIC MODELS OF BRIEF THERAPY

Learning is acquired not to show it off, but to use it.

G. C. Lichtenberg, *The Little Book of Consolation*

The evolution of brief therapy from a general model to models of intervention devised specifically for particular types of problems has developed in great part from empirical-experimental research. This research was carried on over several years on hundreds of patients suffering from similar types of pathology. The use of modern strategic logic also helped in the construction of specific forms of treatment capable of fitting the specificity of recurrent typologies of persistence, as described in Chapter 2.

Therefore, the strategies described in this chapter are based on a careful study of the forms of persistence typically found in different types of pathology, of the most effective tactics and maneuvers used for solving these pathologies, and the style of communication most appropriate for each technique and phase of therapy. Although we use the same strategy in all cases that present the same type of disorder and the same attempted solutions that maintain the problem, we always change the type of communication and the type of therapeutic relationship established with the patient, in response to the uniqueness and originality of each individual human system, situation, and context.

The main difference between this specific technique and the nonspecific techniques of brief therapy is that the former requires us to devise specific, focused, repeatable maneuvers able to produce changes in the specific, redundant forms of persistence typical of the main pathologies. This passage from an operative-cognitive level of logic to a cognitive-operative level has produced a remarkable increase in the efficacy and effectiveness of therapy.

For example, our advanced work on the phobic-obsessive syndrome (Nardone 1996, Nardone and Watzlawick 1993) produced truly surprising results: 87 percent of cases solved (Nardone 1998, Sirigatti 1994, Watzlawick and Nardone 1997). In 81 percent of cases, the symptoms disappeared within the first five sessions, and 47 percent of those patients reported that the symptoms had disappeared already after the first session. Our latest project on specific protocols for treating eating disorders has produced equally gratifying results (Nardone et al. 1999).

This evolution of therapy has had very important consequences in the field of professional training. Therapists in training now have precise guidelines for an entire treatment, from beginning to end, to assist them in their work on the pathologies most frequently encountered in the clinical profession.

Another important aspect is that the application of specific treatment protocols by fifty therapists trained at the Center for Strategic Therapy in Arezzo, Italy, has produced similar rates of efficiency and effectiveness to those obtained by treatments administered directly at the Arezzo center. This shows that structured models of specific treatment are more easily taught and transmitted than the general, nonspecific models.

To clarify this further, I now present some examples of specific strategies for treating particular forms of clinical problems. Because I have presented elsewhere in detailed format the protocols of treatment (Nardone 1991, 1996, 1998, Nardone and Watzlawick 1993), I will limit this presentation to a number of therapeutic maneuvers designed to produce the patient's first emotional corrective experience of the problem. I believe that such experiences are essential to any radical change.

I will describe the tactics and techniques used during the second phase of treatment, the phase of unblocking the symptoms. I have chosen these examples to emphasize the systematic and original aspects of this work. They have been constructed specifically to address the persistence of the problem. The therapeutic intervention follows the structure of the persistence, but reverses its direction, using the force of the pathology to produce change.

This strategy has many things in common with the ancient Chinese art of stratagems, as well as with techniques of rhetorical persuasion. Both these technical fields of knowledge are based on the idea that in order to obtain a quick and effective change, people must be led to change their attitudes of perception and reaction without realizing it. Any tricks employed are not revealed until after the change has occurred. To produce this unconscious "leap," these ancient arts (like our own approach to brief therapy) make use of existing resources already contained within the reality to be changed, by applying specific maneuvers that mobilize these resources into a process that inevitably leads to change.

Indeed, I believe that the art of therapy consists of leading patients to construct a situation in which a change of perceptions and reactions is not only desirable but inevitable.

CASE 1: AGORAPHOBIA
WITH PANIC ATTACKS

This generalized type of phobic disorder is maintained by the attempted solutions of avoidance and asking for help. Persons who suffer from this pathology are constantly avoiding exposure to some presumed danger, to the point that they become unable to do anything by themselves without suffering a panic attack, and thus require the constant presence and assistance of a person they trust.

Our research–intervention on phobic–obsessive disorders (Nardone 1996) has shown that when a patient asks for help and receives it, this attempted solution confirms and nourishes the problem. To interrupt this vicious circle quickly, we have devised a specific, elaborate reframing:

> Well, well, first of all there is something I want you to think about during the coming week. I want you to think that each time you ask for help and receive it, you will simultaneously receive two messages. The first, obvious message is "I love you, help you, and protect you." The second message, which is less obvious but stronger and more subtle is "I help you because you can't make it on your own, because you are sick if left on your own." Please note that I am not asking you to stop asking for help, because you are not capable of not asking for help at this time. I am only asking you to think that every time you ask for help and receive it, you contribute to maintaining and worsening your problems. But please, do not make an effort to avoid asking for help, because you are incapable of not asking for help. Only think that every time you ask for help and receive it, you are helping make things worse.

Thus, we state that the patient's problem undeniably requires help from other people, but that although this help may at first have beneficial effects, it will eventually lead to a worsening of the disorder. We are using fear against fear. But the fear of increasing the severity of the problem is much worse than the single fears that constantly drive the person to ask for help. Every fear is limited by some greater fear. As the Romans used to say: *Ubi major minor cessat* (When the biggest one appears the smallest one disappears.)

We do not directly ask the patient to stop asking for help. Instead, we use a paradoxical type of communication, stressing that the patient is unable to do without help. In other words, we induce the person to act, without directly asking for action.

This prescription is normally given at the end of the first session. By the second session, the patients usually report that they never asked for help during the past week; most times, they even started doing things on their own, realized that nothing bad was happening, and kept at it. They even did things they had been avoiding for a long time, without experiencing any fear.

As in the "butterfly effect" of disaster theory (Thom 1990), a small change sets off a chain of greater changes that eventually lead to the catastrophic event. In this case, blocking the attempted solution of asking for help sets off a series of reactions that lead the person to discover that he or she can live without fear. Since it was first formulated, this maneuver has been applied to over 1,000 patients suffering from agoraphobia and panic attacks. In over 70 percent of these cases, it unblocked the pathology.

After the first important change, a whole series of further therapeutic maneuvers and prescriptions is needed to reach a definitive solution. The almost magical effect of the reframing does not indicate recovery from the disorder; however this first concrete experience starts the process of recovery of the patient's own resources.

The importance of this specific technique is more easily understood in light of the existing clinical literature, which emphasizes the great difficulties encountered in obtaining concrete and effective results in the treatment of agoraphobia and panic attack syndromes.

CASE 2: OBSESSIVE-COMPULSIVE BEHAVIOR

The structure of this pathology is mainly conserved by the patient's efforts to control phobic fixations by performing disparate kinds of protective or propitiatory rituals (washing to remove perceived contamination; repeating mental formulas; unusual, irrepressible behavior, etc.). The following prescription has been developed specifically to break this pathogenic vicious circle: "From now to the next session, every time you perform a ritual, you must perform it five times—no more and no less than five times. You may avoid performing the ritual at all; but if you do it, you must do it exactly five times." As I explained previously, the logical structure of this ostensibly simple prescription helps us "lead the enemy into the attic and remove the ladder"; we gain control over the compulsive symptom by making it voluntary, thus defeating itself. The way the prescription is communicated is very important. The communication is based on a redundantly repeated, hypnotic linguistic assonance and on a posthypnotic message, expressed in a more marked tone of voice.

The structure of this maneuver is: if you do the ritual once, you do it five times. I am the one who tells you how many times to repeat it; thus, I am taking control of your symptom. Then I give you the "injunctive" permission to avoid performing the ritual.

Most obsessive-compulsive patients respond to this prescription by following the prescription literally at first, but then after a few days they suspend the rituals. They usually cannot explain why; they just say, "I got bored doing it five times, so I decided to stop."

In the therapeutic protocol for obsessive-compulsive syndromes, this prescription is preceded by a number of preparatory maneuvers, and is usually followed by other specific prescriptions that help the person maintain the effect of this corrective emotional experience (Nardone 1996). These maneuvers are no less important than the disruptive prescription described here. Their role is to help construct a new balance of perception and reaction that will enable the patient to focus on the task, not on the symptom, until the symptom is defeated.

CASE 3: DEPRESSION

In the case of depression, the most common attempted solution is expressed in the patient's tendency to complain and play the victim, which is met by an encouraging, consoling, and protective attitude on the part of the patient's family and friends. Cases of depression therefore require a specific family-systemic type of intervention. We call in the whole family and give the following prescription:

> From now to the next session, you are going to do something very important. You will all gather together every evening, before or after dinner. Take an alarm clock and set it to ring after half an hour. You will all maintain a religious silence while you [to the patient] will have half an hour to complain as much as you want while they all listen. You will have the opportunity to let them know how unhappy you are, and they must listen in religious silence. When the alarm goes off, STOP: the meeting is adjourned to the following evening. You will avoid any reference to the problem during the day: you have the evening time set aside for that purpose.

In most cases, they return and say: "Yes, he [or she] complained a lot the first few evenings, but after a while he didn't have anything left to complain about." Even more interestingly, the patients usually stopped complaining during the day, and began to spend their time doing other things. The depression was all concentrated into the half-hour.

This is an application of the ancient stratagem of "putting out the fire by adding more wood." As in other disorders, after the first corrective emotional experience, we gradually restructure the patient's modes of perception and reaction and apply other, specific maneuvers to guide the person toward a new, functional personal balance.

CASE 4: PARANOIA AND OBSESSIVE DOUBTS

In this case, the basic dysfunctional attempted solution consists of the patient's efforts to provide reasonable, reassuring answers to unreasonable doubts. The more illogical the doubt, the harder he strives to give it a logical answer. As a result, the patient increasingly becomes ensnared in complicated and painful attempts to give rational answers to irrational problems.

We give these patients the following reframing:

You know, there are no intelligent answers to stupid questions. But the questions come to you, and you cannot stop them. On the contrary, if you try to stop them, more of them will come. The Ancients already knew that to think that you are not thinking is, in itself, an act of thinking. In order not to think, you would have to succeed in not thinking about thinking that you are not thinking. You cannot stop the question, because it will come to you. But you can stop the answer, and if you stop the answer, you will gradually inhibit the question. Since you cannot stop the question by making an effort to do so, my suggestion is that you think that every time you try to answer a stupid question with an intelligent answer, you make the question intelligent and encourage it. Thus, every time you give an answer, you encourage further doubts, and the whole thing will not just continue, it will get worse. So every time you answer a stupid doubt with an intelligent answer, you are feeding the vicious circle. If you think about that, you will be able to stop the answer.

In this case, too, the language structure of the maneuver is based on a hyperlogical but hypnotically confusing dynamic that makes large use of repetition and redundancy. We use it to construct a "reality" in which the force of the obsessive symptom is turned around and directed against itself, as in the ancient stratagem of "muddying the waters to make the fish come up to the surface."

Persons with obsessive doubts initially find it difficult to stop answering, but eventually they succeed. Once the answers have stopped, the obsessive questions are no longer nourished, and decrease until they disappear completely. As a result, the obsessive doubts usually stop after a few days.

CASE 5: VOMITING

Although the vomiting syndrome is based on previous anorexic and bulimic symptoms, this infectious eating disorder has its own characteristics of persistence and requires a specific treatment, different from interventions for anorexia or bulimia (Nardone et al. 1999).

The usual attempted solution that maintains the problem is the effort to reduce or control the ritual of stuffing oneself with food and then vomiting. The only effect of this effort is to increase the ritual so much that it often becomes the patient's main daily activity. Since the irrepressible compulsivity of this disorder comes from the pleasure that the patient derives from the ritual, any intervention based on control or repression will only increase the desire to perform it.

Based on this observation, we have developed a tactic, not for controlling the symptom, but for changing the pleasurable perception that makes the compulsion to eat and vomit so irresistible. In more than 50 percent of cases, we have obtained this by the following prescription:

> So, are you truly ready to do anything to get rid of this demon? Good. From now to the next session, I would not dream of asking you to make an effort not to eat and vomit, because you couldn't do it anyway, so do it as many times as you feel the urge. But you will do it as I tell you. From now until our next meeting, every time you eat and vomit, you will eat, eat, eat . . . the way you love to eat. When you have finished eating, at the time when you usually have to go and vomit, stop. Get a timer, set the alarm for an hour later. Wait an hour, without doing anything, without putting anything else into your mouth. As soon as the alarm sounds, not one minute sooner or later, you will run and vomit.

When the patients return, they usually say; "But you spoiled everything that way, because I don't like it as much as before." Indeed, by breaking up the temporal sequence of the eating-vomiting ritual, we alter its irresistible pleasure. In a brutal but effective analogy, it is as if a person who is having sex, and is about to have an orgasm, were to stop and say, "Wait, I'll stop for an hour and then start again." It just wouldn't be the same.

We usually increase the waiting time from one hour to two hours, and then to three hours. After the three-hour interruption, the patients stop vomiting. Again, we take possession of the symptom by using a therapeutic maneuver that follows its structure, but reverses its direction and leads it to self-destruction.

CASE 6: BULIMIA

The basic attempted solution that maintains the bulimic disorder lies in the patient's effort to control the urge to eat by a whole series of constructions, from dieting to locking food away, or avoiding all tempting situations. As a result, the compulsion to devour food becomes increasingly strong and uncontrollable.

The strategic intervention that we have devised for this type of disorder is essentially based on the same logic as the Chinese stratagem of "putting the fire out by adding more wood." Usually, during the third session, the therapist gives the following prescription: "Choose any one of the thousand diets that you know about, but one that is not too restrictive. Whenever you eat something that is not part of this diet, you will eat it five times. If you eat a piece of chocolate, you have to eat five pieces of chocolate; if you eat a piece of cake, you have to eat five pieces of cake. Either don't eat, or eat five."

The most common effect of this prescription is that people either report that they never ate five portions, because they never ate anything that wasn't in their chosen diet, or that they ate five portions a few times, but strangely didn't feel the usual satisfaction, so they stopped.

CASE 7: BLOCKED PERFORMANCE

Some patients are blocked from carrying out a particular behavior, for example, students become unable to take exams, managers can no longer address a convention, or athletes can no longer compete. The problem usually persists and becomes more complicated when they try to prepare themselves more and better for the performance; as a result, they never feel ready, and they keep avoiding the situation.

Our intervention consists of two prescriptions. The first has the aim of reducing the anxiety of anticipation; the second aims to stop these patients' excessive tendency to control themselves during the performance.

First prescription:

I assume that you have an alarm clock at home, the kind with that annoying sound. Well, every day, at the same time you will take the alarm clock and set it to sound half an hour later. During that half hour, you will lock yourself in a room inside your house, sit in an armchair, and try as hard as you can to feel unhappy by thinking about the test you are going to take. You will concentrate on your worst fantasies regarding your problem. Think that everything will go wrong, that you will give a disgraceful performance. Imagine that your worst fears come true, until you deliberately produce a crisis of anxiety and panic. You will remain in that state for the duration of the half hour. Let yourself do whatever you feel like—cry, scream, curse. As soon as the alarm sounds, turn it off and stop the exercise. Leave the thoughts and feelings you induced behind, go and wash your face, and resume your normal activities.

Second prescription:

You will present yourself at the appointed time and place for the test [or exam, public speech, etc.]. When it is your turn to speak, you will start by saying: "Before I start, I ask you to please bear with me, because I will almost certainly have to stop; I know that I will be overcome by my emotions, and lose the thread of my speech." After this preliminary excuse, you should go ahead, and we'll see what happens.

Usually, people come back and report that their attempts to achieve self-induced unhappiness during their "half-hour of suffering" were unsuccessful. Moreover, the test didn't seem so frightening anymore. As for the test itself, their responses vary. The first kind of response is: "You know, I felt confident, so I didn't need to make the preliminary declaration you told me to make." Or: "I did as you told me, and it calmed me. Someone even asked me afterward if saying that was a rhetorical stratagem."

In both cases, the blockage is overcome because the two prescriptions stop the previous, dysfunctional solutions attempted by the patients. "To let the water flow away instead of building embankments" and "advertising instead of hiding" are the two stratagems that make up this intervention, which is carried out in one session. With appropriate adaptations and variations, this almost "faith-healing" kind of intervention has been applied successfully to students, artists, managers, athletes, and others.

CASE 8: AGORAPHOBIA

The therapeutic intervention that has contributed most to the recognition of my work as a clinician and researcher is undoubtedly the ad hoc prescription designed to unblock severe forms of agoraphobia, sometimes defined as chronic agoraphobia. I believe that this fame is due to the intervention's spectacular and "magical" effect when shown to my colleagues on videotape. The logical structure of this intervention has already been described in Chapter 2 of this book, but it may be useful to illustrate it again, from the perspective of clinical practice.

Patients with severe agoraphobia are those who for years have been unable to go out on their own, even for very short stretches or periods of time. In the third session, after a couple of maneuvers that I have already described (reframing the fear of help and half-hour of worst fantasies), we make the following intervention (Nardone, 1996):

> You will now do something very important. Go to the door and make a pirouette. Open the door, go out and make another pirouette. Walk down the stairs. When you get to the front door, make one pirouette before and one after stepping outside. Turn left and keep walking, making a pirouette every fifty steps, until you get to a fruit store. Make a pirouette, go into the store, and buy the largest and ripest apple you can find. Then walk back here, holding the apple in your hand and making a pirouette every fifty steps, and a pirouette before and after stepping inside the building. I will be waiting for you here.

I have personally administered this prescription to more than 500 patients in the past ten years. No one has ever refused to carry it out.

We construct a suggestive situation where making pirouettes seems magical, and apply the stratagem of "sailing the seas without letting the sky know." We shift the patients' attention away from themselves, toward the bizarre task at hand, so that they carry it out without realizing they are thereby overcoming the fear that had, until then, seemed invincible. After this first, irrefutable, concrete experience, we simply lead the patient through a series of further prescriptions that follow the same logical structure, increasing the length and time of the patient's excursions until his or her personal autonomy has been completely recovered.

For this type of disorder, we have an amazingly high efficacy rate of 93 percent of cases solved in an average of seven sessions. Clearly, this result shows that the passage from general therapeutic models to specific protocols of brief therapy has produced a substantial increase in the efficacy and effectiveness of interventions. Indeed, as will be clear from Chapter 7, results have improved remarkably since we started this new line of clinical research about ten years ago.

6

UNUSUAL CASE EXAMPLES: TALES OF APPARENTLY MAGICAL THERAPIES

What distinguishes truly original minds is not that they
are the first to perceive something new, but that they perceive
things that are old, have always been known and overlooked,
as if they were new.

Friedrich Nietzsche

This chapter narrates a number of unusual clinical cases. They are
drawn from over 3,500 cases treated in the past ten years by Giorgio
Nardone and his colleagues at the Center of Strategic Therapy
(Centro di Terapia Strategica) in Arezzo, Italy.

Some cases include examples of strategies that were later
developed into specific protocols for the treatment of several important disorders (Nardone 1998, Nardone and Watzlawick 1993,
Watzlawick and Nardone 1997). There are also examples of interventions developed specifically for unique cases, which should therefore be considered as pure flashes of creativity. We use a narrative

form rather than present complete transcriptions of videotaped sessions, which are available elsewhere (Nardone 1991, 1996, 1999).

CASE 1: THE NEIGHBORS WANT TO SEE ME NAKED

This is the case of a man who had no intention of going into therapy. Therefore, he was brought into therapy by a sort of beneficial trick. We asked his family to tell him that we needed him in order to help his daughter, who was suffering from depression. This stratagem (inviting a reluctant patient to see a therapist, not for himself, but to help a close relative) is an excellent method for starting an indirect therapy.

This man had a strange form of so-called paranoia with persecution complex. He was convinced that his neighbors secretly observed him with video cameras through the ceiling while he undressed before going to bed. I should mention that this man was no supermodel, but an average-looking man in his sixties. In any case, he had this idea that people watched him undress.

When he first came to see me, we talked about his daughter. Then, at one point, he asked me, "Since we're here anyway, I've been told that you're an expert on strategy. I happen to have a problem with my neighbors. They spy on me with video cameras. It's like a war. Since you're such a strategist, you must tell me some strategies."

I showed myself to be interested in his problem. Without contradicting him or voicing any doubt at all about what he was saying, I asked him what he had done to counteract this aggression on the part of his neighbors. He described his attempted solutions. At first, he moved to a new house every time the problem appeared;

he had done that three times. Finally, just to stay on the safe side, he had moved to a place where the apartment above him was vacant. Things definitely seemed to have improved. But then, as fate would have it, something totally unpredictable happened. Not only did someone move into the apartment above him, but who was this new neighbor? The owner of an optical store that sold video cameras. The man's paranoia returned, stronger than ever, and he decided to take action in his own fashion: "Spy on me, and I will torment you."

So the man started tormenting his new neighbors with threatening phone calls at night. The neighbors called the police. Intimidated by the forces of law and order, the man had to tone down his aggression toward his neighbors, but he thought up another "brilliant" solution. He covered his bed with a canopy of thick, black cloth. As he told me, "At first it seemed to me that I had found a permanent solution. I used to get under the black cloth, undress in bed, and throw my clothes out. In the morning, I got dressed under the canopy so that no one could see me."

But then, watching TV during the Gulf War, he discovered the existence of video cameras that can see through walls. His fixations returned, and he resumed his battle against the neighbors.

After listening carefully to his story, I asked, "But have you considered the fact that there is a method for stopping video cameras on airplanes from detecting and recording images? This method was also used during the war."

"I haven't heard about it. Please tell me," he replied.

I asked, "What can we use to blind someone?"

"A flash—a powerful beam of light," he replied.

"Perfect! If we send out a strong beam of light, the video cameras won't be able to see us! So try this experiment during the next two weeks. Buy some spotlights and install them near your bed.

Turn them on every night before going to bed. You will blind the video cameras."

At our next session, the man told me that, wanting to make sure that the strategy was effective, he had bought architectural spotlights of 300 watts each and installed them on the floor by his bed.

"The first night, I left them on the whole night. And we really put them with their back to the wall. They stopped watching me! The second night, I decided to test how long the effects of our strategy could last, so I kept the spotlights on for an hour. Then I turned them off and kept watch to see if the neighbors were trying to trick me, but they didn't dare! After that, I only kept them on for an hour each night, before going to bed." He added, "Maybe we've won!"

"No," I replied, "you mustn't trust them. The enemy is always deceitful. So for the next two weeks, give them an hour of flashes before going to sleep, even if they don't turn the video cameras on. It's a preventive measure, and you'll show them all your power."

The man followed my instructions. At our next session two weeks later, he told me: "After a few days, I noticed that they had stopped turning on the cameras. I actually think they've removed them, so I stopped flashing."

"But," I insisted: "you still need to be careful. They might reinstall them when you're not expecting it. I recommend that you keep on flashing the lights until we meet again in a few weeks."

He returned after a few weeks, and reported: "We've definitely won. The cameras are gone; they've stopped watching me." Then he added, in a rather subdued tone, "What if I made the whole thing up?"

I looked at him and replied, " Do you think we would have done all we did if it hadn't been true? Please, don't give up now!"

When he returned, after one month, he told me; "You know, I really think I made the whole thing up, and that you, with your strategies, helped me realize it."

This clinical example shows that even such severe disorders as this one can be treated in a short time, and sometimes indirectly, without constructing the idea of a traditional therapy. In this case, the person did not even know that he was the subject of a therapeutic intervention. He asked for help with a problem, almost a "war" between himself and the people who, from his point of view, were persecuting him, while he was actually the persecutor. To circumvent his resistance and lead him to change his perception of reality, we used his own logic and mode of representing reality, and led him through a series of corrective emotional experiences, until he began to doubt his previously inflexible convictions. Finally, he discovered, without any direct suggestion on my part, what kind of a mental trap he had entered, after having escaped it. While respecting his logic, our intervention led to the paradoxical saturation and breaking down of this same logic.

CASE 2: THE ENERGY-DRAINING MAGNET

A colleague sent me a patient with whom she had been unable to make any progress. This was due, she told me, to his "delirious expressions." The patient, a man in his thirties, declared that his problem was a conflicted relationship with a colleague at work. According to the patient, his colleague had a magnetic power that was sucking away the patient's vital energy, leaving him empty and exhausted.

As usual, I focused on his attempted solutions. I asked him how he had tried to stop this from happening, how he had attempted to

fight the problem. He replied that he had tried to "stay tough." Sometimes, he had verbally attacked his colleague, but the latter had always
remained unmoved and had always prevailed in the end, sucking away
his energy. As the reader can imagine, the colleague in question may
well have been intimidated by the patient's attitude, and kept quiet
in order to avoid escalation. However, the patient interpreted his
colleague's reaction as a cold and determined strategy.

After listening to the patient's description of the problem and
his attempts to manage it, I did something that is often useful—I
suggested a metaphorical representation of the situation: "If I understand you correctly, it's as if he had a magnet that attracts your
energy to him; this happens whenever you are near each other."

The patient immediately replied, "Exactly, doctor. He's the
magnet that sucks away."

I replied, "But if he's a magnet, how can we stop a magnet
from attracting energy?"

"We need to use glass!" he exclaimed. "Magnets don't stick
on glass."

"Yes," I replied, "but there are other substances that also work
against magnets. I think we've found a way to fight the magnet.
Between now and when I see you again next week, I'd like you to
find a large cellophane bag. Cellophane is a special kind of plastic.
Make yourself a cellophane suit, and wear it every day under your
clothes. That way, we can prevent the magnet from attracting all
your energy, and you'll be able to get your strength back." The
patient looked at me with a strange smile of satisfaction as we said
good-bye.

The following week, he told me he felt as strong as a lion.
Our plan had worked. His energy had not been sucked away. He
had felt uncomfortably hot in the suit, but the main thing was that
the effects of the magnet had been blocked.

Another no less important effect of the stratagem's "magic" was that when the patient's perceptions changed, he reported that the magnet man seemed to have changed so much that he even felt a bit sorry for him. The patient now perceived his former enemy as a poor, innocuous man, and no longer felt any rage toward him.

At that point, I used a technique that I have already described. I asked the young man to imagine how he would behave toward his colleague if the latter were a fragile and timid person in need of reassurance, and to do something every day as if this were true.

I referred the patient back to my colleague, so that she could proceed with her work. After some time, she reported that he had never expressed any more strange ideas; he had even made friends with the man in question.

In this case, our intervention began with the construction of an invented reality that fit with the patient's pathological representations. We used this reality to introduce a change. The change was made possible by the invented reality, which, during our therapeutic interaction, replaced the original reality presented by the subject. An invented reality produced concrete effects. Readers familiar with the field of logic will see that this process is congruent with the logical models of belief and self-deception. As George Lichtenberg wrote, everything that is believed exists.

CASE 3: A PHOBIA OF MIRRORS

A young university student, a psychology major, was referred to me by a psychotherapist who had been treating him for several years. She asked me whether I might be able to cure this young man's bizarre, debilitating phobia: he lived in fear of being drawn toward

a mirror and slamming his nose into it. He had long required various people to assist him, always ready to intervene in case he was
irresistibly drawn into a mirror. He had removed all mirrors from
his house, except for a small one in the bathroom, and used a diaper at night so that he wouldn't have to go in there. His life was
completely impaired both by his phobia and by the strategies he
was using to protect himself from the phobia.

He arrived at my office escorted by one of his "assistant-
protectors," and described his problem. I avoided asking about his
past, any traumas he might have suffered, or his family structure.
Instead, I asked him to describe in detail what attempts he and
the people around him had made to confront the problem. After
he had described his strategies for protecting his nose against
slamming into a mirror, I looked him straight in the eye and told
him I thought it was strange that he had never thought of one
very simple solution. "If you are afraid of slamming your nose
against a mirror," I said, "all you need to do is use one of those
devices that are specifically constructed for protecting noses against
collisions."

He looked surprised and asked, "What devices?" I answered,
"You know, football and motorcycle helmets aren't just made to
protect the head, but the nose too. You could buy yourself a helmet and wear it as you walk around. Every motorcyclist wears a
helmet, so you could just pretend your motorcycle is nearby. That
way, you could move around freely, and be protected by the helmet. I think that might be a better strategy than those you have
used so far to protect yourself against the mirrors that attract your
nose. So, I suggest that you buy a helmet within the next few days.
Get a sturdy one that fits you well, and then we'll see what happens. I think it might help you."

The young man came back a week later, carrying a nice red helmet. He told me that as soon as he got home from our first session, he had started calling different stores, at first looking for a football helmet, but then, since he couldn't find one, settling for a very light but sturdy motorcycle helmet. Eager to try the experiment, he had gone out alone, taken his car (which he had not done for years), driven to the store, walked in and bought the helmet.

It wasn't until he walked out of the store that he realized he had just done something that he couldn't have done before, and without banging against any mirrors, even though he had passed several of them along the way. So he walked home, carrying the helmet and thinking, "Well, if I get really scared, I'll put it on; otherwise I'll just bring it along for safety. " He had gone out again during the week, always taking the helmet along, but never putting it on. As far as I know, he never wore it, but soon got rid of all the other attempted solutions (the protector-assistants, the nightly diaper, and the total isolation).

After a few months, he realized that, thanks to the new strategy, he had completely vanquished his fear of being sucked into a mirror, so he got rid of the helmet, too.

"To sail the ocean unknown to the sky" is to divert a person's attention away from attempting to control the fear and toward a diverting task, prescribed with the help of suggestion. Without realizing it, the person does something that had seemed impossible until that moment. This practical experience necessarily leads, at least for a moment, to a new perception of the reality that had seemed terrifying until a moment earlier. This inevitably loosens up the rigidity of the phobic perceptive-reactive system and opens the path to the construction of new, alternative representations of reality and, thereby, new behavioral and cognitive modes.

CASE 4: THE OBSESSION OF DOING IT IN ONE'S PANTS

Very often, phobic reactions similar to the panic attack syndrome described in the previous chapter develop from an obsession. If we do not subvert the obsessive dynamic at its roots, we will only obtain superficial changes and observe recurrences of the disorder after a short period of time. It is important that the clinical therapist know how to distinguish phobic reactions based on fear from those based on obsessions. Although the treatment will be similar in some aspects, it will be completely different in others (Nardone 1996). The following is a good example of an obsession that led to a phobic reaction.

An elegant and refined middle-aged man traveled a long way to see me. In overly intellectual and verbose language, he described a grotesque problem and its tragic effects. This famous man had an important position in the arts that frequently required him to perform in public. In the past, he had suffered from colitis. Then he began to fear that he might lose control of his bowels during a performance. This had never actually happened, but the fear that it might led him to take some protective measures.

He consulted several gastroenterologists, who assured him that he had nothing to worry about except for a few minor food intolerances. But, as always with obsessive persons, he had not been satisfied by these reassurances and had continued to search for other possible diagnoses. In the course of his vain search, he developed symptoms of anxiety and a phobic outlook.

The situation escalated to such a degree that, in recent years, this patient had almost retired to a kind of protective isolation, avoiding any public situation where his problem might manifest itself. This was supposed to make him feel safer. Instead, his phobic fixations had increased to such an extent that every time he went out he had to have a restroom nearby, in case of an emergency. He kept a mental map of all the available restrooms in his immediate vicinity. Moreover, he restricted his diet to the few things he was sure he could digest without any problem.

In desperation, he began to rely on massive drug therapy, which had slightly reduced his anxiety but had no effect on his basic disorder. He also saw a number of psychotherapists and dropped them due to a lack of results.

At our first session, he told me that, although a dear friend who knew about my work had suggested that he see me, he was quite skeptical. As I usually do in these cases, I accepted his resistance, and prescribed this diffident attitude as something that would be useful to his therapy.

In our first session, I applied some preliminary maneuvers. From the second session on, the therapy focused on interrupting the patient's two basic attempted solutions that maintained the problem: his obsessive attempt to control the symptom by focusing continuously on his intestines, and his avoidance of any situation he perceived as unsafe, including many foods and places where there were no restrooms available. The fundamental technique was the "worst fantasy," which is similarly applied to other disorders, such as panic, depression, and performance blocks. This technique has developed into a series of successive maneuvers. It begins with the following:

I assume that you have an alarm clock at home, one of those clocks with a particularly annoying ring. Every day, at a specific time that we will presently agree upon, you should set the alarm clock to go off after thirty minutes. During that half hour, you will close yourself in a room in your house, sit in an armchair, and do your best to make yourself feel terrible. Concentrate on your worst fantasies regarding your problem. Think about your worst fears, until you deliberately produce a panic attack. Remain in this state for the whole thirty minutes. As soon as the alarm sounds, turn it off, and stop the exercise. Leave behind the thoughts and feelings you produced, go wash your face, and resume your normal daily activities.

The patient followed this prescription. At the next session, he described his reaction as most unexpected. It is, however, the most usual reaction when we prescribe this task. He had not succeeded in producing any sense of unhappiness or unease, or any crisis of fear and anxiety. He had tried to imagine the worst he could think of, but instead he had had only positive fantasies, and had felt very relaxed every time he performed the exercise. He had even fallen asleep in two instances.

I explained that this was the desired effect, and that after this experience he could start using the same technique, which is based on the logic of paradox, training himself until he had learned to cancel the fear by deliberately exasperating it. Then I gave him the next prescription:

From now until our next session, instead of retiring for half an hour to do our exercise, you will perform it five times a day for five minutes, wherever you are, whoever you may be with, at the following times: 9 A.M., 12 noon, 3 P.M., 6 P.M., and 9 P.M. You will keep an eye on your watch, and for five minutes, wherever you are, you will try as hard as you can to bring on your disorder. Remember, do not isolate yourself. You must perform this task within the normal activities that you are carrying out at those times.

With a frightened look on his face, the man asked, "Are you saying that you want me to do it in my pants in public?"

I replied, smiling, "This may happen, but you have seen proof that if you deliberately try to bring on the disorder, it won't happen. So carry out my prescription. We agreed in our first session that you would do whatever I asked you."

At the following session, for the first time, the patient was smiling when he arrived. He had felt much better during the week. He had not felt bad during the five-minute paradoxical exercises. Moreover, since he had noticed that doing the exercise decreased his fear, he had started to abandon his usual route with the reassuring restrooms nearby.

From then on, the therapy focused on increasing his exposure to risks and boosting his confidence in the technique of removing the fear through bringing it on deliberately. He started practicing this technique in situations when he feared that his disorder might occur.

He reported that, as he reclaimed situations long abandoned because he considered them impossible to sustain, he had at times experienced a spontaneous fear, or thought that his intestines were signaling something, but it had been sufficient to deliberately exaggerate the fear in order to make both the fear and the somatic manifestations disappear.

Within ten sessions, the patient regained complete autonomy and was able to face all his public appearances without feeling the terror of incontinence. He also dared to eat foods that he had previously assumed to be indigestible. He discovered that he could now tolerate and digest even fatty and heavy foods that he had thought he would never be able to eat again.

CASE 5: THE REPETITION
OF MENTAL FORMULAS

Another excellent example of how we can intervene quickly and successfully in obsessive-compulsive disorders is that of a young woman who was a victim of a series of ritualized obsessive thoughts.

Several times a day, before and during certain activities, some of which were ordinary ones, she felt a compulsion to mentally repeat formulas made up of words or numbers. This slowed down all her activities, and had the effect of mentally torturing her, since she considered herself a very rational person and could not accept the idea of being forced to do irrational things.

In cases such as this, we use a paradoxical prescription that ritualizes the ritual, as described in the previous chapter, but a less complex one from the formal and logical point of view. We take possession of the compulsive symptom by transforming it. This usually leads to its self-destruction.

I gave the young woman the following prescription:

From this moment until we meet again, every time you feel like repeating one of your formulas, you must repeat them the opposite way. Say all the repetitions you usually say, but the opposite. For example, if you feel like repeating the word *man*, it becomes *nam*. So you will repeat in your mind "nam, nam, nam . . ." as many times as necessary. If the formula is made up of more words and numbers, the exercise will be more difficult. In any case, you have a well-trained mind, right?"

The following session, the patient told me that the whole thing had been exhausting, but very effective, because after a few days the rituals had diminished, and the day before our session there had only been two episodes, which were immediately inhibited by her performance of the prescribed task.

I simply invited the young woman to treasure what she had learned, that is, "to kill the enemy with his own dagger."

CASE 6: THE MOTHER-DEPENDENT PSYCHIATRIST

A psychiatrist applied to our training program in brief strategic therapy. During his admission interview, it emerged that he had some serious personal problems. Therefore, we did not admit him to the program. He then came to me for help in confronting and solving his difficulties.

In therapy, the psychiatrist was able to clearly articulate the basic problem at the root of his mental instability. He felt that he was a victim of a pathological relationship with his mother, who used emotional blackmail to control him. Whenever she did not hear from him for a few hours, she would get completely drunk. She said she did it to calm her anxiety. Her behavior remained balanced if she saw or heard from him.

The mother also had pathogenic reactions every time the psychiatrist told her he had a girlfriend. She would call him every time he was with his girlfriend, crying and falling into a depressive state that always culminated with a large consumption of hard liquor. The son could not turn off his cellular phone because he feared even more extreme reactions, so the mother was able to reach him at any time during the day, wherever he was.

Considering his age and profession, the situation was hard to believe. The psychiatrist still lived with his mother and father, who was also a victim of the mother's behavior. The patient had never spent a night away from home, never gone on vacation, never brought a woman home. He had a relationship with a woman, but went to great lengths to keep it a secret from his parents.

This was clearly a classical "victim–torturer" relationship, maintained by dysfunctional attempts to stop the situation from deteriorating. By following this course of action, he confirmed his mother's belief that her efforts to control him through emotional blackmail, depression, and alcoholism were effective.

We agreed on the rules of the therapy, which the psychiatrist knew, since he was interested in learning our therapeutic model. I prescribed a maneuver directed at reversing the pathogenic mechanism of communication between mother and son.

> From now until next week, you will beat your mother to the punch. You are going to call her. More precisely, you are going to call her ten times a day—every hour, more or less, and you are going ask: "Mother, are you all right? I've been worried about you, you know." As soon as you get an answer, say good-bye and do the same thing one hour later.

Surprised and amused at this idea, the psychiatrist accepted my suggestion. At our next meeting, he told me that at first his mother had assured him she was fine; then she had started telling him to stop it, and finally become very irritated by his too frequent phone calls. However, his mother had not suffered any type of crisis. In fact, she had told her son several times not to worry about her and to think more about himself and his profession, because he seemed a bit stressed.

We increased the number of phone calls from ten to fifteen per day, with the same formula. As a result, the mother began to insist that her son take more care of himself and stop worrying about her; maybe he should take a holiday and try to get some rest. But I instructed him to persist with the phone calls from early in the morning until late at night. After one month of this treatment, we observed that the mother had no crises of depression or alcoholism, nor did she blackmail him during the whole period. Instead, she became very considerate and kind to him, and repeatedly told him to take better care of himself. She even suggested that he might need a passionate love affair to make him feel better and to stop worrying so much about her.

We then planned his first night away from home, to attend a conference. His mother did not suffer any crisis. In fact, she was proud that her son coped so well on his first night away from home.

From then on, we constantly increased the time spent away from home (as often suggested by the mother herself) and gradually decreased the number of phone calls. The crowning moment of the therapy was when the son told his mother about his relationship with his girlfriend, albeit presenting her as a recent conquest. His mother expressed her great satisfaction, especially since she thought she was the mastermind behind her son's success. She never found out that she had been the subject of an indirect treatment.

This case was an example of "throwing away the brick in order to catch the jade," rather than "throwing away the jade in order to get hit by bricks," as the young psychiatrist had done for many years.

CASE 7 : WE CAN HELP YOU DO IT BETTER

The parents of a young girl came to see me because their daughter refused to come. She said that she certainly did not need therapy, and that the parents should go instead, because they were the ones who really needed it.

The girl suffered from what is (I believe, wrongly) defined as bulimia nervosa that is, an eating pattern that consists of bingeing followed by vomiting. I consider the term bulimia nervosa improper, because our research (Nardone et al. 1999) has shown that this type of disorder has nothing to do with bulimia. In most cases, we are dealing with girls with anorexic tendencies. To them, vomiting is a good way to avoid losing or gaining too much weight, or to lose weight while continuing to eat. But after practicing this technique for some time, it becomes an irrepressible compulsion. It is as if these young women (and sometimes men) were possessed by a demon that makes them binge and purge.

The parents told me that they had tried to limit the damages as much as possible. They tried locking the food away. They tried denying their daughter money for her great quantities of food. This had been useless, however, because when she didn't have money, she would shoplift in supermarkets, so they preferred to give her the money. When they tried hiding the food, she was somehow always able to find it.

So they were completely resigned. Their daughter did not want to be cured. She had recently started spending most of her time eating and vomiting. She rarely left the house. She used to have a boyfriend, but she left him. She used to have a group of friends, but she wasn't seeing them anymore. Moreover, her parents told me, she rarely washed and never brushed her hair. She spent all her time bingeing and purging.

We have developed specific techniques based on our research for this disorder, as well as for anorexia and bulimia. The technique I prescribed to the parents is one of those we use when the daughter does not want to come to therapy.

I think there is a way to treat your daughter without her coming, but it's something that may cause you some sacrifices. However, I feel that you're prepared to go through with it because you have already made such great efforts. What I am about to ask you is not as difficult, but it is a little bizarre. Please consider what I'm asking you seriously.

The parents said, "We're prepared to do anything you ask us, because we've heard that you've treated many cases like this, so we trust you."

My prescription was the following:

> From now until next week, every morning before you go to work I would like you (*to the mother*) to wake up your daughter, not too late but not too early and ask her, "What would you like to eat and vomit today?"

The woman looked at me and said, "Do you mean I really have to ask that question?" I replied,

> Of course, exactly that question. You must ask your daughter, "What would you like to eat and vomit today?" Then I want you to write down the menu. Whatever your daughter asks for. Go out and buy everything she asks for. If your daughter refuses to tell you the menu, I think you know what your daughter usually eats and vomits, so buy big portions of that and then go home and put all the food on the table in your dining room, not the kitchen. Put everything on display in the dining room, get some yellow post-it notes and write: "Food for [her name] to eat and vomit." Remember, no one else should touch that food. It is only for your daughter, only for your daughter's ritual.

The parents looked at me dumbstruck, as if what I had asked them to do was even crazier than their daughter's behavior. The father said, "But that will make her really happy!" "We'll see," I replied.

The parents came back the following week, and told me that their daughter had protested violently when she saw the food on the table, and refused to eat it. In fact, she had taken it away and hidden it in a closet. The mother told me, "So to follow your prescription, I put it all out again and added more food to it. Now we have such a lot of food!"

I smiled, and replied, "Well, we'll send whatever is left over to the children who are starving all around the world."

The mother added, "But the most interesting part is that she has considerably diminished her bingeing. It hasn't stopped, but it has decreased."

"Good," I said. "I feel encouraged by this, and we should continue this way. So, remember (*to the mother*) now you will have to do another thing. Remind your daughter, and you, too (*to the father*), remind her several times a day, that she may eat and vomit, the stuff is all there."

"What? Should we really invite her to do it, now that she's doing it less? What if she starts doing it more?"

"We'll see," I repeated. "Remember to invite your daughter to eat and vomit at least four or five times a day, since you bought all that stuff purely for her pleasure." The parents left, even more shocked than the last time.

The next week they came back and told me that their daughter's symptoms had decreased even further; in fact, she got angry every time they told her to eat and vomit, and asked, "Why are you telling me this?"

"In fact," the mother told me, "do you know what she says, doctor? She says I've spoiled everything. It's not like it used to be. She used to enjoy doing it, but she doesn't enjoy it anymore. In fact, my daughter asked me if she could come and see you, because she would like to stop completely."

When the daughter came to see me, the symptoms had not completely disappeared. However, since they had been considerably reduced, it was relatively easy to continue the therapy until the symptoms were completely extinguished.

CASE 8: THE WALL OF SILENCE

One couple that came to me described their relationship as one of absolute mutual indifference, sexual rejection, poor dialogue, and a silent, reciprocal rage. Considering this merry atmosphere, I first saw the two separately. It emerged, from the individual meetings, that each spouse had accumulated such a great rage toward the other that they were punishing each other with the present indifference. Nevertheless, they both declared that they were permanently bound to one another; it was for that very reason that they could not forgive the wrongs suffered in the past.

The interesting thing for an outside observer is that in this type of couple, each spouse considers the other to be guilty, and himself or herself to be in the right. The resulting interaction is similar to two mirrors, each reflecting the other. It is therefore necessary to intervene in such a way as to loosen this rigid position of apparent detachment on the part of both spouses.

After having seen them separately, I brought them together in my office, and gave them the following prescription to be performed until our next session:

> Every night, before or after dinner, you must dedicate half an hour to this exercise. Go to your bedroom, take an alarm clock, set it to ring after fifteen minutes. You (*to the wife*) will sit down, and you (*to the husband*) will remain standing. You have fifteen minutes to let out all your old resentments and accuse your wife of everything you want. Remember, let out all the worst things you want to say to her. When the alarm sounds, you will stop and change roles. You will sit down, and you will stand. You, too (*to the wife*) have fifteen minutes to tell your husband all the worst things you want to say to him. When the alarm sounds, stop. The whole thing is adjourned till the following evening. The next day, you reverse the

order of who starts first, so that neither of you thinks he or she has the last word.

The couple returned the following week. They told me that they had said terrible things, which neither of them would have expected from the other. Both also told me that this was the first time they had felt free to express all the rage they had accumulated over the years. However, both had been surprised by the fact that they felt more free to express their affection as well as their rage. They had sexual relations for the first time in many months, and this past Sunday they had taken a walk in the hills, something they had not done in many years.

At that point, all I needed to do was suggest that they set aside some time every day, perhaps not as formally as in the exercise I had given them before, to express their negative feelings, allowing each other all the time that was needed. I explained that rage and feelings of accusation are like river waters; the more you try to check them, the more they grow, until they break the embankments and flood everything. Instead of checking our rage, we have to let it flow by channeling it if possible, because in that case, as happened to them, the force of the rage can become a positive resource for reviving feelings and emotions of affection.

CASE 9: THE UNENDING THESIS

A very distinguished man of about forty came to me with a rather unusual problem. For about ten years, he had been unable to write his master's thesis in philosophy. He had received very high grades on all his exams, but had been unable to write any of his thesis.

For the past ten years, he had been working as a manager in a company. His work often required him to write reports. He had no problem with that; in fact, he often received compliments for his ability to focus and articulate important questions clearly.

Concerning his thesis, however, he seemed to find it difficult to start writing because he felt that he needed to have complete mastery over his subject. Unfortunately, he had chosen the philosopher Wittgenstein as his subject, about whom new treatises are continually written. For the past ten years, he had been accumulating new texts to read and consult for his thesis. Finally, he reached the conclusion that he suffered from a psychological block that kept him from facing the rite of passage of earning his degree. After attempting to understand the causes of his problem with a psychoanalyst for about a year, to no effect, he decided to come to me.

After listening carefully, I told him that I too was a great admirer of Wittgenstein, and started to discuss the logical-philosophical positions of this author. Our pleasant conversation continued for a while, until I said,

> I am glad to observe that we have an interest in common, but between now and next week, I would like you to think about what would be the best final sentence of your thesis. I mean the very last line of your dissertation on Wittgenstein. Think about it, write it down and bring it to me. I am very curious to see it.

The man came back the following week with the final sentence of his thesis: "Debts are always paid in advance." I was impressed by his choice of this splendid quotation as the closing sentence of his thesis. "That's really beautiful," I said. "Now I would like you to think about what the last page of your thesis, before this marvelous final sentence, should be like."

He came to the next session with the last page. I read it in front of him and commented on the text, asking him to clarify a few points. He replied that those points would be clarified in the preceding pages. "Very well," I said. "I am very curious to read these previous pages, where I will find your explanations to these conclusions. Bring them next time."

The next time, I received the whole final chapter of his thesis (about ten pages), and again read them in his presence, making comments and asking questions.

Within three months, he had written the whole thesis from the end to the beginning, writing the first sentence of the text last.

This is an example of the usefulness of doing things the opposite way. It was also a stratagem for stopping the mental mechanisms that were leading this patient to block his own performance.

The effort of writing his arguments by reversing the usual order, which was certainly not easy to carry out, diverted his attention from his pathogenic "attempted solution" of writing a perfectly updated work.

A tightrope walker cannot brood while he is walking the tightrope. To write backwards is a kind of tightrope walking in the context of writing and argumentation, which blocks the brooding. As the Tao says, "A full mind coincides with an empty mind."

In all the above cases, the difference between a traditional psychotherapist and the one we have described here is clear. The latter may be seen as a sort of "scientific shaman." He is a shaman because, in his interaction with the patient, he is able to construct realities that have the magical power of leading the patient to change his previous modes of perception and reaction. He is scientific in that many of the techniques described here have been made systematic and repeatable, and their efficacy, efficiency, and predictability can be measured.

We wish to make it clear (if it has not been made clear enough) that, as persons who write and practice the therapies described in this book, we absolutely do not wish to be considered as gurus, but rather as technicians of solutions to human problems—a kind of mechanic who unblocks jammed mechanisms.

We would also like to emphasize that although we have referred many times in this book to mental and behavioral problems by their diagnosis, this should not be considered anything more than an expositive device. The intent is to enable the reader to make direct connections between the situations described and certain definitions that have become common usage.

In our view, all the psychiatric and psychological handbooks for the definition of different pathologies could be encapsulated into one simple definition: "person blocked or trapped in her own constructions of reality." As Goethe wrote, "Things are actually much simpler than one might think, but much more complicated than one might realize."

7

OUTCOME
RESEARCH

> Learning to bear clearly in mind that no one is perfectly happy is perhaps the most direct way to achieve happiness. Of course, no one is perfectly happy, but there are many levels to our suffering; this is illness.
>
> G. C. Lichtenberg, *The Little Book of Consolation*

One of the most frequent criticisms of the brief strategic approach is the lack of data on its results. Researchers involved in the comparative evaluation of the results of various kinds of therapy complain that strategic therapists have never systematically presented their findings. Such criticism suggests that the brief strategic approach seems too miraculous or magical to be considered a repeatable and reliable therapeutic model. Brief strategic therapists have been rightly accused of paying little attention and giving scarce importance to the conventional presentation of their data along the usual lines of psychological and social research. And it is true that the strategists have preferred to give ample space to innovative theoretical perspectives and to the description of sometimes eccentric kinds of therapeutic interventions, which in comparison with other therapeutic procedures can often seem too effective and almost magical.

What might even further astonish an outside observer is the way in which the systemic approach and its strategic evolution—based on a rigorous methodology of observation (the use of video recording, the one-way mirror, observers)—may seem to be inadequate regarding the evaluation and systematic presentation of its results. It could certainly be said that strategic therapy has snubbed the research community's requirements for the presentation of its findings. Few and far between are efforts at systematically presenting the results of strategic therapy, as Weakland and colleagues did in 1974, Fisher in 1984, de Shazer in 1986 to 1994, Nardone and Watzlawick in 1993, DeJoug and Berg in 1995, Nardone in 1996, and Watzlawick and Nardone in 1997.

The disparity between the quantity of literature about the theory and practice of strategic therapy and the lack of published systematic results is mirrored by the absence of direct reference to it in the literature of comparative outcome studies. The few data describing brief strategic therapy either are not taken into account because of their scarcity or are incorporated into the data relative to the results of other therapies, above all cognitive-behavior therapy. (For comparative research on therapeutic results, see Asay and Lambert [1999], Barlow [1993], Garfield [1981], and Sirigatti [1988, 1994].)

In this chapter we evaluate the results of brief strategic therapy conducted with a large and heterogeneous group of patients over an extended period of time.

METHODOLOGICAL CRITERIA

Before presenting and discussing the data, it is important to present the methodological criteria of this inquiry, which will illuminate the epistemological and methodological choices underlying those criteria.

The Concept of Efficacy

The evaluation of the effects or results obtained in therapy is one of the thorniest issues in psychotherapy. Much of the difficulty arises from the different schools of psychotherapy having different criteria for establishing the efficacy of therapy, with the unavoidable consequence of diverse theoretical perspectives, which at times assume opposing positions. For example, a Jungian analyst will see the efficacy of therapy in the achievement of personal individuation, while for a behaviorist it will be the extinction of behavioral symptoms.

These are only two of numerous examples of the conceptual disparity in the objectives of therapy and in the evaluation of the efficacy or inefficacy of treatment. It is understandable that different theories of the human personality also provide for different objectives, and that such differences result in different evaluation methods. Once again, our perceptions and conceptions determine our observations.

It is the specific theoretical formulation of human nature that determines the definition of sane or insane, normal or pathological, and, consequently, the notion of recovery and the goals of therapy. There are many different formulations of recovery and of the efficacy of treatment, but, as Sirigatti notes (1988), there seems to be some agreement in defining a specific treatment as effective when it leads to any of the following:

- Symptom abatement
- Increased ability to work
- Better sexual adjustment
- Improvement in interpersonal relations
- Increased ability to confront common psychological difficulties
- Increased ability to react to daily stress

The brief strategic approach, as illustrated in Chapter 3, is not concerned with a theory that can succinctly describe the concepts of normality and abnormality, or with an all-embracing theory of human nature. Rather, it is tied to the constructivist philosophy of knowledge, which, based on the idea of the irreducibility of human nature and behavior to a single, comprehensive description and explanation, is concerned with the appropriate means of making the individual's relationship with reality more functional. From such a theoretical perspective, the efficacy of therapy is represented by the resolution of the patient's specific problem.

The concept of recovery does not entail a complete absence of problems, but rather the overcoming of a specific problem experienced by the patient in a specific time frame and context of his or her life. Therefore, the evaluation of the effects of strategic therapy can certainly be considered to be in agreement with the criteria listed above, with the caveat that no absolute generalization can be made, and that success or the lack of it will be ascertained in relation to the initial therapeutic objectives. Accordingly, success will involve the solution of the patient's presenting problem and the achievement of goals that were agreed upon at the outset of therapy.

Success or lack of success can have many dimensions; therefore, it is important to consider not only the categories of resolved or unresolved cases, but also those relative to cases that are considerably improved or little improved, and it is also crucial to evaluate the possibility of deterioration following the end of therapy (Asay and Lambert 1999, Sirigatti 1988, 1994). The criteria for establishing efficacy used in this evaluative inquiry are defined below. To evaluate the efficacy of the treatment, we used two sets of parameters. One is the effectiveness of the treatment (the evaluation of the outcome of therapy). Were the goals that the patient and therapist agreed upon at the beginning of therapy achieved? Were the patient's problems resolved at the end of therapy? Was there a shift in the original symptom? The second is the efficacy of treatment over time. Were the results of therapy maintained over time, or was there a relapse? Have new problems replaced the original ones?

Three follow-up sessions were arranged for three months, six months, and one year after the end of treatment. The follow-up sessions were conducted as interviews directly with the patient and his family or partner, Many authors use phone follow-up (de Shazer 1985, Geyerhofer and Komori 1995, Talmon 1990).

We consider a case resolved and the treatment completely successful only when, in addition to fulfilling the first set of parameters, the second set of parameters is also fulfilled, that is, when the disappearance of symptoms and problems at the end of therapy is maintained over time, without relapses or substitution of new symptoms for the original ones.

The evaluation of the effects of therapy is based on five categories of results:

1. *Resolved cases*: complete resolution of the problem at the end of therapy and absence of relapses within one year.

2. *Considerably improved cases:* complete remission of symptoms at the end of therapy, but with subsequent sporadic and slight relapses.

3. *Somewhat improved cases:* partial remission of symptoms at the end of therapy, with occasional crises and recurrence of the symptoms reported at follow-up. However, such problems were generally described as being considerably less serious than those before therapy.

4. *Unchanged cases:* treatment accomplished no significant change in the patient's situation after ten sessions. In these cases, treatment ended after the tenth session because there was reason to believe that continuation was not likely to produce change.

5. *Worsened cases:* treatment led to a worsening of the patient's condition.

Beyond defining and measuring efficacy, it is important to evaluate it in relation to the nature of the patient's problems. For a sound evaluation of the efficacy of a therapeutic model, one must take note of the type of problem the model confronts with greater or lesser efficacy (the efficacy differential).

The data presented here are grouped into seven categories. The evaluation of efficacy, in addition to being applied to the entire sample, was also differentiated in regard to the types of problems treated. The definition—at times ambiguous—of the problem or disorder was made through consideration of the patient's prevalent or dominant symptoms. The classifications are as follows:

- Anxiety disorders, phobias, and panic
- Obsessions and obsessive-compulsive disorders
- Sexual problems

- Relational problems
- Depressive disorders
- Eating disorders (anorexia, bulimia, and vomiting)
- Psychoses or supposed psychoses

This empirically based set of categories is in keeping with the *DSM-IV* classifications of psychiatric diagnostic standards for all disorders except for relational problems, which, perhaps because they are purely relationship problems, are not included in the manual.

It is important, nevertheless, to remember that the systemic and strategic approach avoids the traditional nosological and psychiatric classifications, insofar as they hardly take into account the complexity of human systems. We prefer to speak of problem typologies and their solutions. The classification presented here, apparently contradicting these traditional epistemological positions, was chosen with a view toward establishing a frame of reference that is not strictly limited to the systemic approach. We believe that this is the only way of allowing comparisons between the results of this therapeutic model and others.

This subdivision of problem typologies, based on the cases treated from January 1988 to September 1998 at the Strategic Therapy Center (Centro di Terapia Strategica) in Arezzo, Italy, can be considered a balanced cases study, because of the large and varied sample (3,985 cases).

The Concept of Cost-effectiveness

After having established good results regarding efficacy, the second relevant aspect of therapy is its cost-effectiveness (Garfield 1980). This aspect has great theoretical and social importance; in fact, there is quite a significant cost difference between the solution of a problem in three months and a solution in three years. The difference is not only in the cost, but also in the fact that a person is going to live better and more happily as soon as the problems that led him to therapy are solved. But oddly enough, as Garfield (1980) notes, what would seem to be a fundamental rule of professional ethics—the speedy solution of problems and suffering—has not been much considered by psychotherapists. Garfield explains this apparently incomprehensible attitude with the fact that for decades psychotherapeutic thought has been dominated by the idea that, to be effective, therapy must be prolonged, deep, and complex. However, this view, typical of traditional psychotherapeutic theories, has been decisively refuted by research on the comparative efficacy of psychotherapy. In fact, the data clearly demonstrate that there are no significant differences between results obtained in long-term therapy and those obtained in shorter therapy (Avnet 1965, Bloom 1995, Butcher and Koss, 1986, Garfield et al. 1971, Gurman and Kniskern 1986, Harris et al. 1963, 1964, Luborsky et al. 1975, Phillips and Wiener 1966, Schlien 1957, Sirigatti 1994). In some cases, the research even indicated that shorter-term therapy was more effective (Bloom 1995, Nardone 1996).

This position is confirmed by Asay and Lambert (1999):

> The beneficial effects of therapy can be achieved in short periods (5 to 10 sessions) with at least 50% of clients seen in routine clinical practice. For most clients, therapy will be Brief. This is not meant to be an endorsement of Brief therapy. It is simply a statement of fact. In consequence, therapists need to organize their work to optimize outcomes within a few sessions. Therapists also need to develop and practice intervention methods that assume clients will be in therapy for fewer than 10 sessions. A sizable minority of clients (20% to 30%) requires treatments lasting more than 25 sessions. [p. 24]

Careful consideration of cost-effectiveness should be an important factor in the analysis and evaluation of the power of a therapeutic model. The amount of time committed to obtaining a result qualifies the result itself; in fact, the relation between therapy's costs and benefits will be more positive the less prolonged the treatment.

To measure the cost-effectiveness of our work, we utilized a breakdown similar to that used to present efficacy (see Figure 7–4). Cost-effectiveness was measured in terms of the median duration of treatment, both at the general level and at the differential level by type of disorder. In addition, cost-effectiveness was judged by setting aside from the total sample all cases with positive outcome: the completely resolved cases and those considerably improved (see Figure 7–3).

Evaluation of our results leads us to several conclusions, about both the capacity of this specific interventive model and general themes of therapy evaluation.

THE SAMPLE

The sample (Figure 7–1) comprises all cases treated at the Center of Strategic Therapy (Centro di Terapia Strategica) in Arezzo, Italy, from January 1988 to September 1998. Since the center is a private clinic, the patients came for treatment of their own accord, and in that sense they represent a random sample. The only variables that all patients share are the request for therapy at the same center and the fact of being treated with strategic therapy.

The sample comprises 3,484 cases, including 436 persons who had originally requested therapy (12 percent) but abandoned therapy during the first three sessions and were considered dropouts). The sample is 42 percent male and 58 percent female, with a median

Figure 7–1: Sample distribution—classes of pathologies.

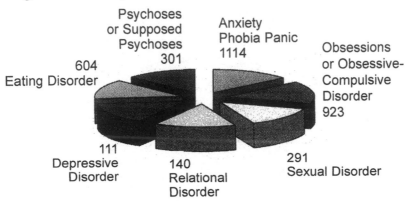

age of 26 (range, 6 to 71). The social standing and professional activities of the patients are quite disparate and heterogeneous.

RESULTS

General Success

The efficacy of this type of treatment is clearly demonstrated in its high general success rate. The positive outcomes of treatment are 86 percent of the treated cases (Figure 7–2). In addition, this efficacy is even more evident in regard to specific problems, such as phobic disorders (agoraphobia and panic attacks), where there is a success rate of 95 percent (Figure 7–3) (Nardone 1996). If we compare these data with the results in the literature on the efficacy of different psychotherapeutic approaches (Andrews and Harvey 1981,

Figure 7–2: Treatment efficacy.

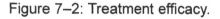

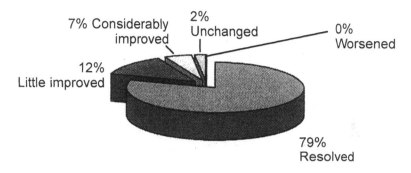

7% Considerably improved

2% Unchanged

0% Worsened

12% Little improved

79% Resolved

Total cases: 3,640   86% with positive effect

Barlow 1993, Bergin and Strupp 1972, Garfield 1981, Giles 1983, Luborsky et al. 1975, Sirigatti 1988, Strupp and Hadley 1979), which estimate the positive success rate of various therapies, according to the various approaches and research data, at 50 percent to 80 percent , it is obvious that the strategic approach has an efficacy superior to the other approaches. It also passed the follow-up test one year after the end of therapy.

Success Over Time

The treatment efficacy of the strategic approach is maintained over time. The percentage of relapses is quite low, and the results obtained at the end of therapy are maintained in the majority of cases through the third follow-up, after one year—making future relapses or the emergence of substitute symptoms rather unlikely. In accord with Garfield (1980) and Asay and Lambert (1999), this

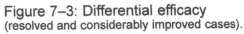

Figure 7–3: Differential efficacy
(resolved and considerably improved cases).

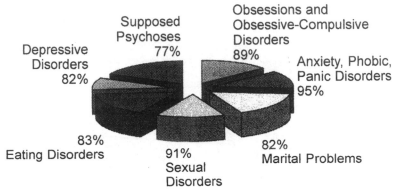

refutes the supposition, common among many therapists, that short-term therapies are superficial and lead inevitably to relapses into the original problem (or symptom displacement).

Treatment Effectiveness

Treatment effectiveness is the characteristic that, we believe, distinguishes the results of strategic therapy from those of other approaches. There is obviously quite a difference between therapy that lasts (on average) nine sessions and one that lasts 835 (the average duration of psychoanalytic treatments in the Menninger Foundation Psychotherapy Research Project, as reported by Garfield 1981) (Figure 7–4). The real cost of the longer or shorter duration of therapy is not, it seems to us, primarily economic, but rather its bearing on the patient's quality of life. The difference between the successful treatment of a severely agoraphobic patient in seven sessions (three or four months) or in 150 sessions (three or four years) is that in the former the patient feels considerably better after only a few months, whereas in the latter the patient must continue to live for quite a long time dominated by this problem. Referring again to Garfield (1980) and Asay and Lambert (1999), it seems crucial to establish which therapy will best serve a given patient's needs with the least expense, either economic or emotional. Therapy must begin with these concerns in mind, but if these procedures are not working or prove to be inadequate, it is then legitimate to move on to other procedures that might prove to be more effective. Of course, not all human problems can be solved in a brief time, but, to be sure, one must try.

Once a specific form of therapy has shown its efficacy, its cost-effectiveness becomes a factor of major consideration. If it is neces-

Figure 7–4: Duration of treatment: whole sample.
(Median duration of therapy: 9 sessions)

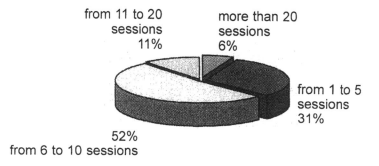

from 11 to 20 sessions 11%

more than 20 sessions 6%

from 1 to 5 sessions 31%

52% from 6 to 10 sessions

sary to use manipulative strategies or "beneficial confusion"—as in
many of the cases described in this book—we maintain that such
tactics are the most correct and ethical insofar as the goal is to help
the patients solve their problems as quickly as possible. Therefore,
manipulation and beneficial confusion are not instruments of tor-
ture, but strategies to break down patients' resistance to change, and
thus lead to their feeling better with the least emotional and economic cost.

Finally, if we consider the results obtained by advanced forms
of brief strategic therapy when applied specifically to particular problems (as we have done in the past decade), we see that the both the
efficacy and the effectiveness of this approach have increased, com-
pared with the already satisfactory results obtained by the previous
general models (Figure 7–5). This increase in efficacy has been

Figure 7–5: Effectiveness of treatment.
(Median duration of therapy for resolved and considerably improved
cases: 7 sessions)

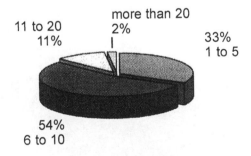

around 10 percent: from an average efficacy of 70 to 75 percent until the mid-1980s (Gurman and Kniskern 1986, Gustafson 1986, Butcher and Koss 1986, Weakland et al. 1974, to 80 to 86 percent in the following ten years (Bloom 1995, de Shazer 1985, Geyerhofer and Komori 1995, Monteczuma 1996, Nardone 1996, Nardone and Watzlawick 1993), with high points of efficacy reaching above 95 percent for particular forms of disorders (Madanes 1990, 1995, Nardone 1996).

In terms of effectiveness, the number of sessions necessary to obtain the solution of the patient's presented problems has decreased to an average of five or six sessions (Bloom 1995, de Shazer 1991, 1994, Geyerhofer and Komori 1995, Watzlawick and Nardone 1997), with the mobilizing of symptoms increasingly starting during the first few sessions, and often after the first session (Bloom 1995, Nardone 1998, Talmon 1990).

If we compare these results with those of different forms of evolved psychotherapy (Asay and Lambert 1999, Sirigatti 1988, 1994), we find that brief strategic approaches are unquestionably better at reaching more effective solutions to most mental and behavioral disorders at a lower cost (financially and emotionally).

Initially, brief therapy depended on the intuitions of the therapists. But brief therapy has become a rigorous model, based on continuous technical advancements developed from empirical clinical practice, applied research, and the most advanced theoretical and epistemological formulations.

The eighteenth-century scholar George Lichtenberg's statement that the "best proof of a theory lies in its application" remains true even in this fascinating and too often mysterious field of knowledge. The same is true for Gregory Bateson's assertion that "there is nothing more practical than a good theory."

EPILOGUE

As T.S. Eliot wrote, at the end of the journey we find that we are back at the starting point. Indeed, after this long, complex journey through the universe of brief strategic therapy, we must return to our opening statement that brief strategic therapy is an original approach to the formation and solution of human problems, which has its own theoretical and epistemological foundations and its own specific procedures of application, whose constant evolution is based on empirical research.

This approach offers no "truths", only "keys" to the solution of problems. Dogma and orthodoxy are replaced by knowledge and awareness. After all, as Gregory Bateson stated, the task of science is to construct solutions for specific problems.

According to ancient Zen Buddhism, there are two types of truth: truths of essence and truths of error. The first type can only be reached through enlightenment; at that point, one no longer belongs to this world, because "essence" is "transcendence". The second type of truth is "instrumental", useful for constructing and carrying out projects in the world of objects and appearances. Each truth of error is shattered after being used, and must be replaced by other "truths of error" suitable for the varying circumstances faced by living beings. The strategic approach concerns itself with truths of error that enable human beings to better manage their realities.

REFERENCES

Alexander, F. (1956). *Psychoanalysis and Psychotherapy*. New York: Norton.

Alexander, F., and French, T. M. (1946). *Psychoanalytic Therapy*. New York: Ronald Press.

Andrews, G., and Harvey, R. (1981). Does psychotherapy benefit neurotic patients? A reanalysis of the Smith, Glass, and Miller data. *Archives of General Psychiatry* 38:1203–1208.

Anonimo. (1990). *I 36 stratagemmi: l'arte cinese di vincere*. Napoli: Guida Editori.

Asay T. P., and Lambert M. J. (1999). The empirical case for the common factors in therapy: quantitative findings. In *The Heart and Soul of Change,* ed. M. A. Hubble, B. L. Duncan, and S. D. Miller. Washington DC: American Psychological Association.

Ashby, W. R. (1954). *Design for a Brain*. New York: Wiley. [*Progetto per un Cervello.*] Milano: Bompiani, 1970.

———. (1956). *An Introduction to Cybernetics*. London: Methuen. [*Introduzione alla Cibernetica.*] Torino: Einaudi, 1971.

Austin, J. L. (1962). *How to Do Things with Words*. Cambridge, MA: Harvard University Press. [*Come Fare Cose con le Parole*. Genova: Marietti, 1987.]

Avnet, H. H. (1965). How effective is short-term therapy? In *Short-Term Psychotherapy*, ed. L. R. Wolberg, New York: Grune & Stratton.

Balint, M. (1968). *The Basic Fault*. London: Tavistock.

Bandler, R., and Grinder, J. (1975a). *Patterns of the Hypnotic Technique of Milton H. Erickson, M.D.* Palo Alto, CA: Meta.

————. (1975b). *The Structure of Magic*. Palo Alto, CA: Meta.

Barlow, D. F. (1993). *Clinical Handbook of Psychological Disorders, 2nd ed.* New York: Guilford.

Bartlett, F. C. (1932). *Remembering: A Study in Experimental and Social Psychology*. Cambridge, England: Cambridge University Press.

Bateson, G. (1961). *Perceval's Narrative—A Patient's Account of His Psychosis, 1830–1832*. Stanford, CA: Stanford University Press.

————. (1967). Cybernetic explanation. *American Behavioral Scientist* 10(8):29–32.

————. (1972). *Steps to an Ecology of Mind*. New York: Ballantine. [*Verso un'Ecologia della Mente*. Milano: Adelphi, 1976.]

————. (1979). *Mind and Nature: A Necessary Unity*. New York: Dutton. [*Mente e Natura*. Milano: Adelphi, 1984.]

Bateson, G., and Jackson, D. D. (1964). Some varieties of pathogenic organization. In *Disorders of Communication*, ed. D. McK. Rioch, pp. 270–283 Washington, DC: Research publications, vol. 42. Association for Research in Nervous and Mental Disease.

Bateson, G., Jackson, D. D., Haley, J., and Weakland, J. H. (1956). Toward a theory of schizophrenia. *Behavioral Science* 1:251–264.

Berg, I. K. (1985). Helping referral sources help. *Family Therapy Networker* 9(3):59–62.

————. (1994). *Family-Based Services: A Solution-Focused Approach*. New York: Norton.

Berg, I. K., and de Shazer, S. (1993). Wie man Zahlen Zum Sprechen bringt: Die Sprache in der Therapie. *Familiendynamik* 1:51–56.

Bergin, A. E., and Strupp, H. H. (1972). *Changing Frontiers in the Science of Psychotherapy*. Chicago: Aldine.

Bergman, J. S. (1985). *Fishing for Barracuda—Pragmatics of Brief Systemic Therapy*. New York: Norton.

Berkeley, G. (1710). *A Treatise Concerning the Principles of Human Knowledge*. Parts 1 and 3. [*Trattato sui Principi della Conoscenza Umana*. Bari: Laterza, 1984.]

Bertalanffy, L. von (1956). General system theory. *General Systems Yearbook* 1:1–10.

———. (1962). General system theory—a critical review. *General Systems Yearbook* 7:1–20.

Bloom, B. (1995). *Planned Short-Term Therapy*. Needham Heights, MA: Allyn & Bacon.

Brown, G. S. (1973). *Laws of Form*. New York: Bantam.

Butcher, J. N., and Koss, M. P. (1986). Research on brief and crisis-oriented therapies. In *Handbook of Psychotherapy and Behavior Change: An Empirical Analysis*, ed. S. L. Garfield, and A. E. Bergin, 3rd ed. New York: Wiley.

Cade, B., and O'Hanlon, W. H. (1993). *A Brief Guide to Brief Therapy*. New York: Norton.

Cialdini, R. B. (1984). *Influence: How and Why People Agree to Things*. New York: Morrow.

Da Costa, N. (1989a). On the logic of belief. *Philosophical and Phenomenological Research* 2:35–56.

———. (1989b). The logic of self-deception. *American Philosophical Quarterly* 1:11–29.

DeJong, P., and Berg, I. K. (1998). *Interviewing for Solutions*. Forrest Lodge, CA: Brooks-Cole.

De Man, P. (1979). *Allegories of Reading*. New Haven, CT: Yale University Press.

de Shazer, S. (1975). Brief therapy: two's company. *Family Process* 14:79–93.

———. (1982a). *Patterns of Brief Family Therapy*. New York: Guilford.

————. (1982b). Some conceptual distinctions are more useful than others. *Family Process* 21:79–93.

————. (1984). The death of resistance. *Family Process* 23(1):11–17, 20–21.

————. (1985). *Keys to Solution in Brief Therapy.* New York: Norton. [*Chiavi per la Soluzione in Terapia Breve.* Roma: Astrolabio, 1986.]

————. (1988a). *Clues: Investigating Solutions in Brief Therapy.* New York: Norton.

————. (1988b). Utilization: the foundation of solutions. In *Developing Ericksonian Therapy: State of the Art,* ed. J. K. Zeig and S. R. Lankton, pp. 112–124. New York: Brunner/Mazel.

————. (1991). *Putting Difference to Work.* New York: Norton.

————. (1993). Creative misunderstanding: there is no escape from language. In *Therapeutic Conversations,* ed. S. Gilligan and R. Price, pp. 81–90. New York: Norton.

————. (1994). *Words Were Originally Magic.* New York: Norton.

de Shazer, S., and Molnar, A. (1984). Four useful interventions in brief family therapy. *Journal of Marital and Family Therapy* 10(3):297–304.

Dini, V. (1980). *Il Potere Delle Antiche Madri* (*Maternal Power in Ancient Times*). Turin, Italy: Boringhieri.

Elster, J. (1979). *Ulysses and the Sirens.* Cambridge, England: Cambridge University Press.

————. ed. (1985). *The Multiple Self.* Cambridge, England: Cambridge University Press and Universitetfarlaget AS (Norwegian University Press).

Epston, D. (1993). Internalizing discourses versus externalizing discourses. In *Therapeutic Conversations,* ed. S. Gilligan and R. Price, pp. 161–177. New York: Norton.

Erickson, M. H. (1952). Deep hypnosis and its induction. In *Experimental Hypnosis,* ed. L. M. LeCron, pp. 70–114. New York: Macmillan.

————. (1954a). Special techniques of brief hypnotherapy. *Journal of*

Clinical and Experimental Hypnosis 2:109–129. In *Opere*, vol. 4, ed. M. H. Erickson, pp. 179–206. New York: Irvington.

———. (1954b). Pseudo-orientation in time as a hypnotic procedure. *Journal of Clinical and Experimental Hypnosis* 2:161–283. In *Opere*, vol. 4, ed. M. H. Erickson, pp. 449–475. New York: Irvington.

———. (1958). Naturalistic techniques of hypnosis. *American Journal of Clinical Hypnosis* 1:3–8.

———. (1964). The confusion technique in hypnosis. *American Journal of Clinical Hypnosis* 6:183–207. In *Opere*, vol. 1, ed. M. H. Erickson, pp. 288–326. New York: Irvington.

———. (1965). The use of symptoms as an integral part of hypnotherapy. *American Journal of Clinical Hypnosis* 8:57–65.

———. (1980). *The Collected Papers of Milton H. Erickson on Hypnosis,* vol. 1–4, ed. E. L. Rossi. New York: Irvington.

Erickson, M. H., and Rossi, E. L. (1975). Varieties of double bind. *American Journal of Clinical Hypnosis* 17:143–157. In *Opere*, vol. 1, ed. M. H. Erickson, pp. 469–489. New York: Irvington.

———. (1977). Autohypnotic experiences of Milton H. Erickson. *American Journal of Clinical Hypnosis* 20:36–54.

———. (1979). *Hypnotherapy: An Exploratory Casebook.* New York: Irvington.

———. (1983). *Healing in Hypnosis.* New York: Irvington.

Erickson, M. H., Rossi, E. L., and Rossi, S. I. (1979). *Hypnotic Realities: The Induction of Clinical Hypnosis and Forms of Indirect Suggestion.* New York: Irvington.

Fisch, R., Weakland, J. H., and Segal, L. (1982). *The Tactics of Change: Doing Therapy Briefly.* San Francisco: Jossey-Bass.

Fisher, S. G. (1984). Time-limited brief therapy with families: a one-year follow-up study. *Family Process* 23(1):101–106.

Foerster, H. von. (1970). Thoughts and notes on cognition. In *Cognition: A Multiple View,* ed. P. L. Garvin. New York: Plenum.

———. (1973). On constructing a reality. In *Environmental Design Re-*

search, vol. 2, ed. W. F. E. Preiser, pp. 35–46. Stroudsburg: Dowden, Hutchinson and Ross.

———. (1974a). Notes pour une éspistemologie des objets vivants. In *L'unité de l'homme*, ed. E. Morin and M. Piattelli-Palmarini. Paris: Le Seuil.

———. (1974b). Kybernetik einer Erkenntnistheorie (Cybernetic Epistemology). In *Kybernetik und Bionik* (*Cybernetics and Bionics*), ed. W. D. Kcidel, W. Handler, and M. Spring. Munich: Oldenburg.

———. (1981). *Observing Systems*. Seaside, CA: Intersystems.

———. (1984). On constructing a reality. In *The Invented Reality*, ed. P. Watzlawick, pp. 51–64. New York: Norton.

———. (1991). Las semillas de la cibernética. (The cybernetic evolution: invented ideas.) In *Obras Escogidas*, ed. M. Pakman, pp. 9–11. Barcelona: Gedisa.

Frank, J. D. (1973). *Persuasion and Healing*. Baltimore, MD: Johns Hopkins University Press.

Frankl, V. E. (1960). Paradoxical intention. *American Journal of Psychotherapy* 14:520–535.

Freud, S. (1993). New introductory lectures on psycho-analysis. *Standard Edition* 22:5–182.

Garcia T., and Witzaele, J. J. (1993). *L'Ecole du Palo Alto*. Paris: Edition du Seuil.

Garfield, S. L. (1978). Research on client variables in psychotherapy. In *Handbook of Psychotherapy and Behavior Change: An Empirical Analysis*, ed. S. L. Garfield and A. E. Bergin, 2nd ed. New York: Wiley.

———. (1980). *Psychotherapy: An Eclectic Approach*. New York: Wiley.

———. (1981). Psychotherapy: a 40 years appraisal. *American Psychologist* 2:174–183.

Garfield, S. L., Prager, R. A., and Bergin, A. E. (1971). Evaluation of outcome in psychotherapy. *Journal of Consulting and Clinical Psychology* 37(3):307–313.

Geyerhofer, S., and Komori, Y. (1995). Bringing forth family resources in therapy. *Zeitschrift für Sozialpsychologie und Gruppendynamik* 20(3).

Giles, T. R. (1983). Probable superiority of behavioral interventions. I: traditional comparative outcome. *Journal of Behavioral Therapy and Experimental Psychiatry* 14:29–32.

Glasersfeld, E. von. (1979). Cybernetic experience and concept of self. In *A Cybernetic Approach to Assessment of Children: Towards More Humane Use of Human Beings,* ed. M. N. Ozer. Boulder, CO: Westview Press.

———. (1984). An introduction to radical constructivism. In *The Invented Reality,* ed. P. Watzlawick. New York: Norton.

———. (1995). *Radical Constructivism.* London: Falmer.

Glover, E. (1956). *Freud or Jung?* New York: Meridian.

Grana, N. (1990). *Contraddizione e Incompletezza. (Contradictions and Incompleteness).* Napoli: Liguori.

Greenberg, G. (1980). Problem-focused brief family interactional psychotherapy. In *Group and Family Therapy,* ed. M. D. Wolberg, L. Marvin, and P. D. Aronson, pp. 112–134. New York: Brunner/Mazel.

Gurman, A. S. (1981). Integrative marital therapy: toward the development of an interpersonal approach. In *Forms of Brief Therapy*, ed. S. Budman, pp. 51–70. New York: Guilford.

Gurman, A. S., and Kniskern, D. P. (1986). Research on marital and family therapy. In *Handbook of Psychotherapy and Behavior Change: An Empirical Analysis,* ed. S. L. Garfield and A. E. Bergin, 3rd ed. pp. 192–221. New York: Wiley.

Gustafson, J. P. (1986). *The Complex Secret of Brief Psychotherapy.* New York: Norton.

Haley, J. (1963). *Strategies of Psychotherapy.* New York: Grune & Stratton. [*Strategie della Psicoterapia.* Firenze: Sansoni, 1985.]

———. (1967). *Advanced Techniques of Hypnosis and Therapy: Selected Papers of Milton H. Erickson, M.D.* New York: Grune & Stratton. [*Le Nuove Vie dell'Ipnosi.* Roma: Astrolabio, 1978.]

———. (1973). *Uncommon Therapy: The Psychiatric Techniques of Milton H. Erickson, M.D.* New York: Norton. [*Terapie non Comuni.* Roma: Astrolabio, 1976.]

————. (1976). *Problem Solving Therapy*. San Francisco: Jossey-Bass. [*La Terapia del Problem Solving*. Roma: La Nuova Italia Scientifica, 1985.]

————. (1982). The contributions to therapy of Milton H. Erickson, M.D. In *Ericksonian Approaches to Hypnosis and Psychotherapy*, ed. J. K. Zeig, pp. 5–25. New York: Brunner/Mazel.

————. (1984). *Ordeal Therapy. Unusual Ways to Change Behavior*. San Francisco: Jossey-Bass.

————. (1985). *Conversations with Milton H. Erickson M.D.* Vol. 1: *Changing Individuals*, Vol. 2: *Changing Couples*, Vol. 3: *Changing Families and Children*. Washington, DC: Triangle.

Harris, M. R., Kalis, B., and Freeman, E. (1963). Precipitating stress: an approach to brief therapy. *American Journal of Psychotherapy* 17:465–471.

————. (1964). An approach to short-term psychotherapy. *Mind* 2:198–206.

Heisenberg, W. (1958). *Physics and Philosophy*. New York: Harper.

Herr, J. J., and Weakland, J. H. (1979). *Counseling Elders and Their Families: Practical Techniques for Applied Gerontology*. New York: Springer.

Hubble M. A., Duncan B. L., and Miller S. D. (1999). *The Heart and Soul of Change*. Washington. DC: American Psychological Association.

Hugo, V. (1862). *Les Misérables*. New York: American Publishers.

Jackson, D. D., and Weakland, J. H. (1961). Family therapy: some considerations on theory, technique, and results. *Psychiatry* 24 (suppl. 2):30–45.

Jakobson, R. (1963). *Essais de Linguistique Generale* (*Essays in General Linguistics*). Paris: Editions de Minuit.

Jones, R. A. (1974). *Self-Fulfilling Prophecies*. New York: Halsted.

Korzybski, A. (1933). *Science and Sanity: An Introduction to Non-Aristotelian Systems and General Semantics*. Lancaster, England: International Non-Aristotelian Library.

Koss, M. (1979). Length of psychotherapy for clients seen in private practice. *Journal of Consulting and Clinical Psychology* 47(1):210–212.

Kuhn, T. (1970). *The Structure of Scientific Revolutions*. Chicago: University of Chicago Press.

Laing, J. (1970). *Knots*. New York: Pantheon.

Luborsky, L., Singer, B., and Luborsky, L. (1975). Comparative studies of psychotherapies: Is it true that everyone has won and all must have prizes? *Archives of General Psychiatry* 132:995–1004.

Macdonald, A. J. (1994). Brief therapy in adult psychiatry. *Journal of Family Therapy* 16(4):415–426.

Madanes, C. (1981). *Strategic Family Therapy*. San Francisco: Jossey-Bass.

———. (1984). *Behind the One-Way Mirror*. San Francisco: Jossey-Bass.

———. (1990). *Sex, Love and Violence*. New York: Norton.

———. (1995). *Violence of Man*. San Francisco: Jossey-Bass.

Mahoney, M. J. (1991). *Human Change Processes*. New York: Basic Books.

Mally, E. (1926). *Grundgesetze des Sollens (Basic Laws of Moral Obligations)*. Graz, Austria: Leuscher & Lubenky.

Maturana, H. R. (1978). Biology of language: the epistemology of reality. In *Psychology and Biology of Language and Thought,* ed. G. A. Miller and E. Lennberg. New York: Academic Press.

Maturana, H. R., Uribe, G., and Frenk, S. G. (1968). A biological theory of relativistic colour coding in the primate retina. *Archivos de Biologìa y Medicina Experimentales* Suppl. 1:1–30.

Maturana, H. R., and Varela, F. J. (1980). *Autopoiesis and Cognition: The Realization of the Living*. Dordrecht, Holland: Reidel. [*Autopoiesi e Cognizione*. Venezia: Marsilio, 1985.]

Mayo, E. (1933). *The Human Problems of Industrial Civilization*. New York: Macmillan.

Monteczuma, C. (1996). Speech presented at *Global Reach of Brief Therapy*, held at Vienna nel Giugno. [*Evaluation of brief therapy results*.] Presented at the Congress "The Global Reach of Brief Therapy," Vienna, June.

Morin, E. (1985). Le vie della complessità. In *La Sfida della Complessità*, ed. G. Bocchi and M. Cerutti. Milano: Feltrinelli.

————. (1993). *Introduzione al Pensiero Complesso*. Milano: Sperling e Kupfer.

Moscovici, S. (1967). Communication processes and properties of language. In *Advances in Experimental Social Psychology*, vol. 3, ed. L. Berkowitz, pp. 225–270. New York: Academic Press.

————. (1972). *The Psychosociology of Language*. Chicago: Markham.

————. (1976). *Social Influence and Social Change*. New York: Academic Press.

Nardone, G., ed. (1988). *Modelli di Psicoterapia a Confronto (Confrontational Psychotherapy)*. Rome: Il Ventaglio.

————. (1991). *Suggestione –> Ristrutturazione = Cambiamento. (Suggestions, Reframing, Change). L'approccio Strategico e Costruttivista alla Psicoterapia Breve*. Milano: Giuffrè.

————. (1995). Brief strategic therapy of phobic disorders: a model of therapy and evaluation research. In *Propagations: Thirty Years of Influence from the Mental Research Institute*, ed. J. H. Weakland and W. A. Ray. New York: Harworth.

————. (1996) *Brief Strategic Solution-Oriented Therapy of Phobic and Obsessive Disorders*. Northvale, NJ: Jason Aronson.

————. (1998). *Psicosoluzioni. (Psychosolutions)*. Milano: BUR.

Nardone, G., Milanese, R., and Verbitz, T. (1999). *Le Prigiani del Cibo: Vomiting, Anoressia, Bulimia. Fireure:* Ponte alle Grazie (*Escaping from the Prisons of Food*, published in English).

Nardone, G., and Watzlawick, P. (1993). *The Art of Change*. San Francisco: Jossey-Bass.

Pascal, B. (1962). *Pensieri*. Torino: Einaudi.

Phillips, D. (1974). The influence of suggestion on suicide: substantive and theoretical implications of the Werther effect. *American Sociological Review* 39:340–354.

————. (1979). Suicide, motor vehicle fatalities, and the mass media: evidence toward a theory of suggestion. *American Journal of Sociology* 84:1150–1174.

————— (1980). Airplane accident, murder, and the mass media: toward a theory of imitation and suggestion. *Social Forces* 58:1001–1024.

Phillips, E. L., and Wiener, D. N. (1966). *Short-Term Psychotherapy and Structural Behavior Change*. New York: McGraw-Hill.

Piaget, J. (1937). *La Construction du Réel Chez l'Enfant*. Paris: Delachaux et Niestlé, Neuchâtel. [*La Costruzione del Reale nel Bambino*. Firenze: La Nuova Italia, 1973.]

—————. (1954). *The Construction of Reality in the Child*. New York: Basic Books.

—————. (1970). *Genetic Epistemology*. New York: Columbia University Press.

—————. (1971). *Biology and Knowledge*. Chicago: University of Chicago Press.

Popper, K. R. (1972). *Objective Knowledge*. London: Oxford University Press. [*Conoscenza Oggettiva. Un Punto di Vista Evoluzionistico*. Roma: Armando, 1979.]

—————. (1983). *Realism and the Aim of Science*. London: Hutchinson.

Prigogine, I. (1980). *From Being to Becoming*. San Francisco: Freeman.

Rosenthal, R. (1966). *Experimenter Effects in Behavioral Research*. New York: Appleton-Century-Crofts.

Rosenthal, R., and Jacobson, L. (1968). *Pygmalion in the Classroom: Teacher Expectation and Pupils' Intellectual Development*. New York: Holt, Rinehart & Winston. [*Pigmalione in Classe*. Milano: Angeli, 1983.]

Salvini, A. (1988). Pluralismo teorico e pragmatismo conoscitivo: assunti metateorici in psicologia della personalità. In *Pluralismo Teorico e Pragmatismo Conoscitivo in Psicologia della Personalità*, ed. E. Fiora, I. Pedrabissi, and A. Salvini. Milano: Giuffrè.

—————. (1995). Gli schemi di tipizzazione della personalità in psicologia clinica e psicoterapia. In *Nuove Prospettive in Psicoterapia e Modelli Interattivo-Cognitivi*, ed. G. Pagliaro and M. Cesa-Bianchi. Milano: Angeli.

Salzman, L. (1968). Reply to critics. *International Journal of Psychiatry* 6:473–476.

Schimmel, A., ed. (1983). *Die Orientalische Katze* (*The Oriental Cat*). Cologne: Diederichs.

Schlien, J. M. (1957). Time-limited psychotherapy: an experimental investigation of practical values and theoretical implications. *Journal of Counseling Psychology* 4:318–329.

Schopenhauer, A. (1912). *Über den Willen in der Natur*. Munich: Piper. [*La Volontà della Natura*. Bari: Laterza, 1973.]

Schrödinger, E. (1958). *Mind and Matter*. Cambridge, England: Cambridge University Press.

Simon, F., Stierlin, H., and Wynne, L. (1985). *The Language of Family Therapy: A Systemic Vocabulary and Sourcebook*. New York: Family Process Press.

Sirigatti, S. (1988). La ricerca valutativa in psicoterapia: modelli e prospettive (The evaluative research in psychotherapy). In *Modelli di Psicoterapia a Confronto*, ed. G. Nardone. Roma: Il Ventaglio.

———. (1994). La ricerca sui processi e i risultati della psicoterapia (The research on the processes and the results of psychotherapy). *Scienze dell'Interazione* 1(1):117–130.

Spencer Brown, G. (1969). *Laws of Form*. London: Allen & Unwin.

Stolzenberg, G. (1978). *Can an Inquiry into the Foundations of Mathematics Tell Us Anything Interesting About Mind?* New York: Academic Press.

Strupp, H. H., and Hadley, S. W. (1979). Specific versus nonspecific factors in psychotherapy: a controlled study of outcome. *Archives of General Psychiatry* 36:1125–1136.

Talmon, M. (1990). *Single Session Therapy*. San Francisco: Jossey-Bass.

Thom, R. (1990). *Parabole e Catastrofi*. *(Catastrophes and Parables)*. Milano: Il Saggiatore.

Vaihinger, H. (1924). *The Philosophy of "As If,"* trans. C. K. Ogden. New York: Harcourt Brace.

Varela, F. J. (1975). A calculus for self-reference. *International Journal of General Systems* 2:5–24.

———. (1979). *Principles of Biological Autonomy.* New York: North Holland.

Watzlawick, P. (1964). *An Anthology of Human Communication: Text and Tape.* Palo Alto, CA: Science & Behavior Books.

———. (1976). *How Real is Real?* New York: Random House.

———. (1978). *The Language of Change.* New York: Basic Books.

———. ed. (1984). *The Invented Reality.* New York: Norton.

———. (1985). Hypnotherapy without trance. In *Ericksonian Psychotherapy, vol. 1, Structure,* ed. J. Zeig. New York: Brunner/Mazel.

———. (1990). Therapy is what you say it is. In *Brief Therapy: Myths, Methods and Metaphors,* ed. J. K. Zeig and S. G. Gilligan, pp. 55–61. New York: Brunner/Mazel.

Watzlawick, P., Beavin, J. H., and Jackson, D. D. (1967). *Pragmatics of Human Communication. A Study of Interactional Patterns, Pathologies and Paradoxes.* New York: Norton.

Watzlawick, P., and Nardone, G. (1997). *Terapia Breve Strategica (Brief Strategic Therapy).* Milan: Raffaello Cortina Editore.

Watzlawick, P., and Weakland, J. H., eds. (1977). *The Interactional View.* New York: Norton.

Watzlawick, P., Weakland, J. H., and Fisch, R. (1974). *Change: Principles of Problem Formation and Problem Solution.* New York: Norton.

Weakland, J. H. (1993). Conversation—but what kind? In *Therapeutic Conversations,* ed. S. Gilligan, and R. Price. New York: Norton.

Weakland, J. H., Fisch, R., Watzlawick, P., and Bodin, A. M. (1974). Brief therapy: focused problem resolution. *Family Process* 13(2):141–168.

Weakland, J. H., and Ray, W. A., eds. (1995). *Propagations: Thirty Years of Influence from the Mental Research Institute.* New York: Haworth.

Whitehead, A. N., and Russell, B. (1910–1913). *Principia Mathematica.* Cambridge, England: Cambridge University Press.

Wiener, N. (1967). *The Human Use of Human Beings: Cybernetics and Society,* 2nd ed. New York: Avon.

————. (1975). *Cybernetics, or Control and Communication in the Animal and the Machine,* 2nd ed. Cambridge, MA: Massachusetts Institute of Technology Press.

Wittezaele, J. J., and Garcia, T. (1992). *A la Recherche de L'école de Palo Alto.* (*The Palo Alto School's Research*). Paris: Le Seuil.

INDEX

ABOUT THE AUTHORS

Dr. Giorgio Nardone is the Director of the Centro di Terapia Strategica and of the Post Graduate School of Brief Strategic Therapy in Arezzo, Italy. He is also Professor of Brief Psychotherapy at the Post Graduate School of Clinical Psychology, University of Siena, Italy. With a Ph.D. in educational science from the University of Siena, where for five years he has been a researcher at the Institute of The Science Philosophy on the epistemology of the psychotherapy models, he also received the title of Specialist in Clinical Psychology at the School of Medicine, University of Siena.

Dr. Nardone has published many articles and eleven books, translated into several languages, including *The Art of Change,* with Paul Watzlawick, and *Brief Strategic Solution-Oriented Therapy of Phobic and Obsessive Disorders.* His systematic and effective models in treating phobic, obsessive-compulsive, and eating disorders are utilized by psychotherapists throughout the world.

Giorgio Nardone regularly conducts conferences and workshops in both Western and Eastern countries, as well as at his Institute in Arezzo.

Paul Watzlawick, Ph.D., has been a research associate at the Mental Research Institute of Palo Alto, California, since 1960. Much of the work of the Institute is based on his endeavors, and MRI is well-known throughout Europe and South America because of his publications and frequent appearances at universities and psychotherapy conferences. MRI "residents," students from around the world who train here, have been introduced to the Institute by Dr. Watzlawick.

His original training was at the C. G. Jung Institute at Zurich. From 1957 to 1960 he held the Chair of Psychopathology and Psychotherapy at the National University of El Salvador (Central America).

Dr. Watzlawick is clinical professor emeritus at the Department of Psychiatry and Behavioral Sciences, Stanford University Medical Center, and visiting professor at the University of Valparaiso (Chile). His many honors include: *doctor honoris causa* at the University of Liege (Belgium), Bordeaux-III (France), Buenos Aires (Argentina), and Webster University (Vienna, Austria).

Fluent in German, Italian, Spanish, and French, Dr. Watzlawick is author or co-author of eighteen books, in 87 foreign language editions, and 141 book chapter or articles in professional journals.

Dr. Watzlawick also consults with major U. S. and international corporations and is expanding the community outreach programs at MRI, bringing his work and MRI resources to business.